H2O Workouts

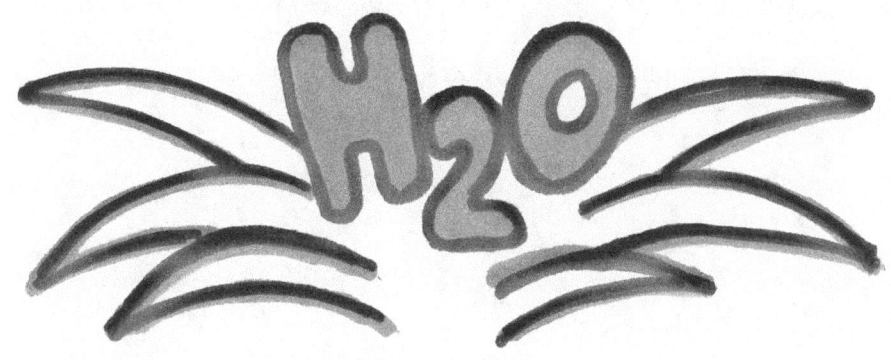

Basic Water Workout

By Francine Milford

H2O Workouts: Basic Water Workout

By Francine Milford

ISBN: **978-1-4357-2289-7**

Photographs by Paul Milford

Caution

The techniques, ideas, and suggestions presented in this book are not intended as a substitute for proper medical advice. Any application of the techniques, ideas, and suggestions in this book is at the reader's sole discretion and risk.

Table of Contents

Chapter One

Fitness for the Next Generation

As more people are recognizing the need to live healthier and better lives, they have begun to set goals on how they will achieve and maintain a healthy body through proper nutrition and balanced work schedules. More than ever before, physical fitness is playing a vital role in helping them to achieve their goals. With full support and encouragement from many family physicians, family members are told to go out and exercise at least three days a week.

Gyms and exercise studios began to spring up all over the country and many forms of physical exercise were introduced. Who can forget the Jane Fonda workout videos and the Jack Le lane television spots?

Step Reebok joined the group offering a twist to the standard floor aerobics by adding a bench to the class format. Soon, balls, slides, and weights were added to the typical exercise class.

Floor aerobics began to add dance movements such as in Hip Hop, Dancercise and Jazzercise routines. Marital art moves such as Qigong and Tai Chi were also added to the classic aerobic studio classes, as well as, boxing and kickboxing.

Before long, the entire face of a typical aerobic class was changed as millions of people attempted to find a way to add exercise into their daily lives. Classes ranged in levels from easy senior workouts and classes for pregnant women to the high paced, high intensity Boot Camp classes.

Soon, many people were experiencing injuries from pushing their bodies too long and too far. When people are impatient to see results, they tend to exercise for long hours in a short period of time. Over use injuries is one of the most common injuries found in the fitness industry, and no one is immune from the dangers of injury.

As baby boomers are entering the fitness world for the first time, they find their choice severely limited due to their own health and physical fitness levels. The fitness industry began to change again to welcome this largest group of exercisers to hit the gym facilities ever.

Now most facilities offer Tai Chi, Qigong, Yoga and Pilates for people who want a good workout without the stress and strain of strenuous exercise.

A word of caution for those who are entering a Yoga class for the first time, find an instructor who is experienced in handling first time attendees and can direct you into moves for your fitness level. Be sure to let your instructor know of any physical limitations or problems you may have before class begins so that they can help guide you during the exercises. This is very, very important.

I have personally seen many first time class participants become injured in a yoga class by attempting to do movements that their bodies were not ready to do.

If it feels wrong, chances are the moves are wrong for you. Don't ever allow yourself to be coaxed or threatened into a move that doesn't feel right for you. Speak up and don't be shy. After all, if you are injured, you will be the one suffering for your mistake-not the instructor.

For people who have gone the route listed above and are still looking for an exercise program in addition to walking and bicycling, the water has become very popular.

I call the water environment, the Great Equalizer. When I have taught water aerobic classes I would have ladies enter the water on crutches and even one came to class in a wheelchair. Once in the water, you could not tell the ladies apart. In the water environment, everyone is equal and everyone can receive a workout that is right for them and their fitness level.

And for those who doubt, one former student told me after class, "I didn't know you could sweat in the water." Don't let the soft and serene look of the water fool you. You can achieve a workout in the water that is equal to any on land. You get out of your workout what you put into a workout.

In this book I will be sure to list exercises in **LEVELS**. If you are a beginner, then please stick to **Level One** exercises. As your body becomes familiar with the moves and becomes stronger, then move on up to **Level Two** and **Level Three**. Remember, don't over due your workouts or you risk injuring your body and not being able to exercise at all. I would rather see you do a short ten minute workout everyday to build yourself up to the half hour or hour workout.

Be sure to get the approval of your primary health care physician before beginning this or any exercise routine.

Principles of Water Exercise

The water environment offers two important natural occurring effects to the water routine: buoyancy and resistance.

Buoyancy is the property of being able to float. Buoyancy is also the power of a liquid to keep objects afloat; in this case, that object is you.

It is the natural ability of water to act as a cushion and in so doing, it protects you joints from injury, strain and reinjury. Many rehabilitation centers use the water environment in their treatment sessions.

While in the water environment, people can perform exercises they otherwise could not on land. Among these exercises are jumps, leaps, jumping jacks and pivots.

Amazingly enough, the ability of water to be buoyant also allows water to provide resistance to water aerobics. Through changing direction, adding speed, or using longer levers, the water can provide a complete and thorough workout.

The water environment can become a natural total body workout. The more you put into your workout, the more you will receive from it. The faster you move, the harder the exercise becomes. Water aerobics provide a safe alternative to the land aerobic class.

Water aerobics is also the perfect environment for those who are overweight or suffer from physical injuries. When you stand in water that is chest deep, you weigh only 10% of your normal body weight.

In water where you cannot touch the bottom of the pool, you will receive a total non impact workout. (Be sure to wear a flotation device if you are planning on deep water exercises.)

The water environment is also the great place to practice your golf or tennis swing. Even dancers and weight trainers can use the resistance in the water to build up muscles in a safe way.

There are now many books and tapes out on the market that will can help you with your water workout, or check out the selection available at your local library.

Preparing to get Wet

When beginning your water exercise routine, the most important consideration is your swim suit. Find a suit that will cling comfortably to your body and still allow you freedom of movement.

Stay away from suits that will quickly fill with water with each jump that you take or that will ride up with each kick. If a suit isn't comfortable you will be fussing more with the suit than you will be concentrating on the exercises.

Don't skimp when making your swimming suit purchase. A good suit should last you the entire season without falling apart. Think ahead and purchase your suit at the end-of-season clearance rack.

The second consideration is what to wear on your feet. Not everyone will be comfortable in wearing something on their feet while doing exercises in the water.

The bottom of the pool may be harsh on your feet through consistent movement. I haven't always had problems with this happening to my own feet, but it has happened, especially in backyard pools.

You have plenty of choices to make when selecting what to wear on your feet. A pair of socks with good elastic is always an inexpensive purchase. I use a white booty sock that you will see later on in pictures in this book. I also own a pair of water socks (light shoes designed for walking in water) and a pair of water shoes. Yes, they actually look like tennis shoes but are made to go from land to water. I wear these shoes when I teach water aerobics as they add the perfect cushion for performing the moves on land.

There are also hand gloves, water buoys and pool noodles available to add resistance to your water workout. Many department stores and retail outlets now sell these products to water exercise enthusiasts.

I highly suggest that you hold off on purchases until you have already begun your water workouts and find out whether or not you need more of resistance training, then make you purchase.

Developing your Wet Workout

Do's and Dont's

- Do wear aqua shoes, or aqua socks, that are comfortable.
- Do keep head in alignment of the spine.
- Do exercise in water that is of correct depth to you and the exercises that you are performing.
- Do relax and breathe slowly and deeply.
- Drink plenty of water before, during, and after your exercise routine.
- Consult with your doctor before beginning this or any other exercise program.
- Work at your own fitness level. You are NOT in competition with anyone else but yourself.
- Stop exercising if you feel faint, dizzy, nausea, or shortness of breath.
- Don't smoke or drink alcohol while doing these or any other exercises.
- Don't make fast, uncontrolled movements of the head or trunk in any direction.
- Don't use extreme range of motion.
- Don't use quick, jerky movement. Everything should flow slowly and smoothly together.
- Don't exercise with food or gum in your mouth.
- If you feel tired-stop

Tips for a Safe Workout

For your safety, there should be a lifeguard on duty during your water workout. If there is no lifeguard present, consider using the 'buddy system' and invite a friend to exercise with you.

Never drink alcohol before, during, or immediately after a water workout. Alcohol can impair your sense of balance, judgment and coordination.

Perform your exercises in water that is chest high. Be sure you have enough room to extend your arms straight from your body without hitting the sides of the pool, or another swimmer.

Wait at least 1-3 hours after eating before working out in the water, longer if your workout is going to be more strenuous.

When you enter the water that is cool, be sure to beginning walking, jogging, or bouncing right away to get your circulation moving.

Always begin your exercising slowly and then working up to more strenuous, energetic moves after your muscles have been warmed up to prepare them for it.

If you feel tired, light headed, or dizzy, stop immediately and ask for help.

Keep a bottle of water within easy reach for a quick refreshing gulp when you need it.

Keep a large towel handy to wrap yourself in and dry yourself off with for after you get out of the pool. Try to stay away from drafts or cold breezes if possible.

Remember-Have fun!

Your Target Heart Rate

Your target heart rate is the highest your pulse rate can get, or should get. When you work within your target heart rate you can be assured that you are receiving a good cardiovascular workout. But this may not be good for everyone.

If you are on medication to lower your heart rate, or have a medical condition such as high blood pressure, heart disease or diabetes, then you should certainly contact your health care provider to ask for advice on what your target heart rate should be. Working at a greater intensity level than what is safe for you could cause serious side effects. Please talk this over with your doctor.

To calculate your Target Heart Rate:

220 – Your Age = Predicted Maximum Heart Rate

Example: A 50 year olds predicted heart rate is 170.

220 – 50 = 170

****

Now that you have discovered your maximum heart rate, this is the rate you should never go over. **Most people work within 60% to 85% of their target heart rate.**

If you were the 50 year old used in the example above with a predicted heart rate of 170, you would work within the 60% to 85% of your heart rate which would be between **102** and **145**.

There is no need to ever exercise beyond 85% of your target heart rate. Doing so would increase both the chances of cardiovascular and orthopedic risk while doing nothing to increase any benefits to your body. See the chart on next page for easy reference:

Chart for Target Heart

Age	Target Heart Rate (HR) Zone (60-85%)	Predicted Maximum Heart Rate
20	120-170	200
25	117-166	195
30	114-162	190
35	111-157	185
40	108-153	180
45	105-149	175
50	102-145	170
55	99-140	165
60	96-136	160
65	93-132	155
70	90-128	150

Like other aerobic exercise, participants want to achieve their maximum heart rate in order to improve the capacity of the cardio respiratory system. Exercise in water is no different. Below is a simple formula to follow to estimate your **Pulse Rate.**

Your pulse rate is your heart rate. It is the number of times that your heart beats in one minute. At rest, you will notice that your heart, or pulse, rate is lower than when you are active. Pulse rates vary from person to person and depend upon a lot of different factors such as age and physical fitness of the individual.

Knowing how to take your pulse rate can you ensure that you are receiving a proper cardiovascular workout (if that is your goal). It may be difficult at first to find and read your pulse, but with practice, it will become second nature.

When taking your pulse, you will use the second and third fingers of your dominant hand. You will place these fingers at your choice of three separate locations: The Temple, the Carotid Artery in the neck, and the wrist. Practice these positions and find the one that is easiest for you to locate the pulse on:

1. Your Temple

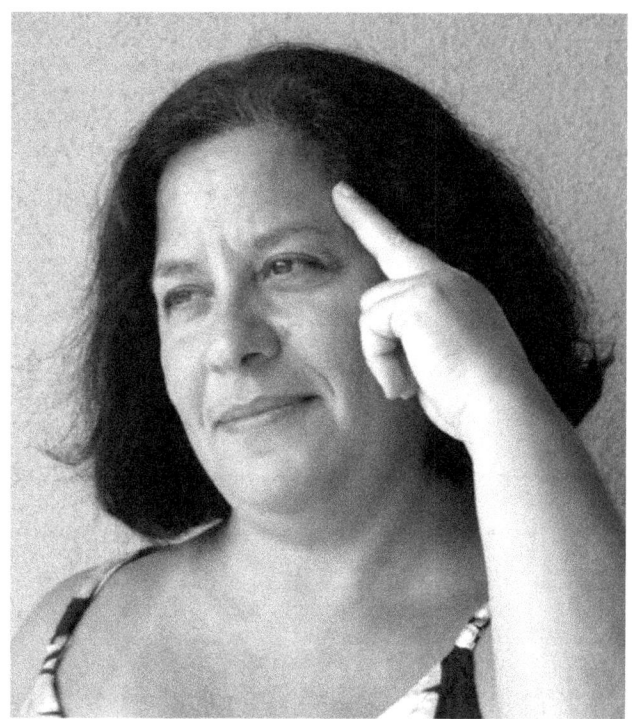

2. The Carotid Artery in your Neck

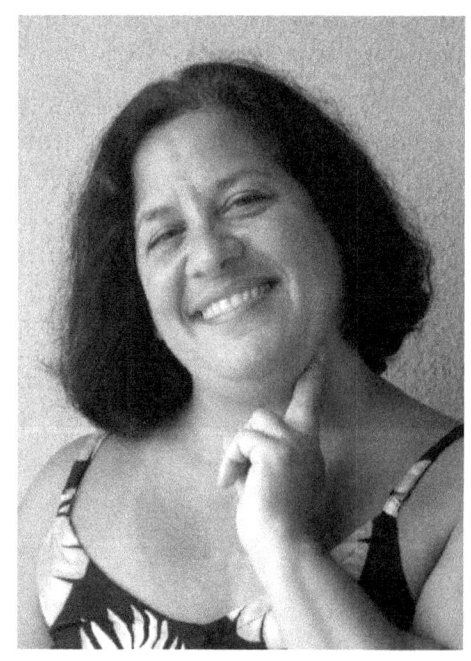

3. Your Wrist

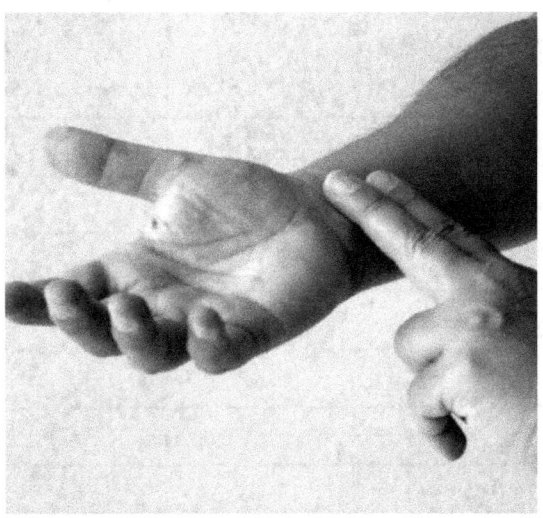

To Do:

Place the second and third finger of your dominant hand at the area you have chosen. For most people, the Carotid Artery in the neck is the place where it is easiest to locate the pulse.

You should also have a clock, or watch, with a second hand available to watch the seconds.

You will place your fingers gently on the area you have chose and count the beats that you feel for 10 seconds. This is your beginning pulse rate. Halfway through your workout you will stop and take your pulse rate again to be sure you are working within your correct heart rate chart. At the end of your workout and cool down, you will take your pulse rate one last time to be sure that you have allowed enough time for your body to return to a pre-aerobic state.

In the water environment, we count the beats that you feel for 6 seconds, rather than the 10 seconds we use on land. Research has found that body cools down a lot faster in the water environment than on land.

A normal pulse rate for children ages six to fifteen is 70-100 beats per minute. For adults over the age of 18, a normal pulse rate is 60-100 beats per minute.

Laminated Heart Rate Charts are available from www.fwonline.com and cost about $19.95 plus postage and handling.

Two simple and easy charts to follow are shown below:

10 Second Chart to Determine Intensity of Workout on Land

AGE in YEARS	50%	60%	70%	80%
50	14	17	20	23
55	14	16	19	22
60	13	16	19	21
65	13	16	18	21
70	12	15	18	20
75	12	14	17	19
80	12	14	16	18
85	11	14	15	18
90	11	13	15	17
95	10	12	15	17
100	10	12	14	16

6 Second Chart to Determine Intensity of Workout on Land

6 sec. HEART RATE

Age	60%	70%	75%	80%	85%
20	11	13	14	15	16
25	11	13	14	14	15
30	11	12	13	14	15
35	10	12	13	14	15
40	10	12	12	13	14
45	10	11	12	13	14
50	9	11	12	12	13
55	9	11	11	12	13
60	9	10	11	12	12
65	8	10	11	11	12
70	8	10	10	11	12
75	8	9	10	10	11

Chapter Two

Warm-ups

As in any exercise program, it is important to prepare the body for the work that you are planning to put it through. We call this preparation, the Warm-Up.

In the Warm-Up you will increase the flow of blood to each and every muscle of the body. In this way, you will greatly reduce the risk of injury.

Warm-up exercises are usually gentle and slow activities that normally last 5 to 15 minutes. During this phase all the muscles and joints should be put through simple movements beginning with small range of motions and then increasing to larger, or full, range of motion.

In a typical land aerobic or workout class, we begin simply with marching in placing. The same holds true for water aerobics. In this chapter we will include several muscle groups that you will need to be sure you warm-up before beginning a water aerobic class. For some, this may be all the exercise that you can do in one day and if so, that is perfectly okay. What is important is move and stretch your body as often as you can throughout the day to keep it limber and lubricated.

When I received my certification in Aquatic Exercise, we practiced many types of water walking. Following a 3 to 5 minute warm-up exercise (such as marching in place) you could do some of the following walking exercises for the next 20-45 minutes:

- Walk forward and backwards
- Walk to the right and Walk to the left
- Walk in a big clockwise circle, then walk in a big counter clockwise circle
- Walk on your toes
- Walk on your heels
- Walk like a crab sideways bouncing from flat feet with knees bent and open to the sides of your body.
- Walk forward and backward while your punch the water.
- Walk three steps and hop for one step.
- Do the Congo line step in the water.
- Do the Bunny hop in the water.
- Do the Electric Slide in the water.
- Do your favorite Western Two Step in the water.
- Alternate between fast and slow walking to add intensity.
- Do the Soldier Walk, otherwise known on Goose Stepping
- Do Karate Kicks
- Walk doing knee lifts forward and front leg lift backwards
- Do Pendulum Swings with your legs side to side

- Do the Rocking Horse forward and backwards and change legs.
- Do Hamstring Curls forward and backwards.

When stretching muscles in the warm-up phase it would be good if you could hold each stretch for at least 10 seconds (30 seconds is optimal).

When performing the warm-up exercises and stretches, you should be able to feel slight warmth within your body. This is good and signals that you are preparing your body for the more vigorous workout that is to follow.

The muscles that are stretched during the warm-up phase are the muscles that will be worked through the aerobic phase.

The Toe and Ankle Warm-ups

Some warm-up exercises and stretches can be performed inside, or at poolside, before you ever enter the water. If you find it difficult to spend more than 20 minutes in the water, then performing the warm-up stretches before entering the water may be a good idea.

Remember, do the best that you can but don't push your body beyond its physical limitation and most of all – Have Fun!

1. Toes and Ankles

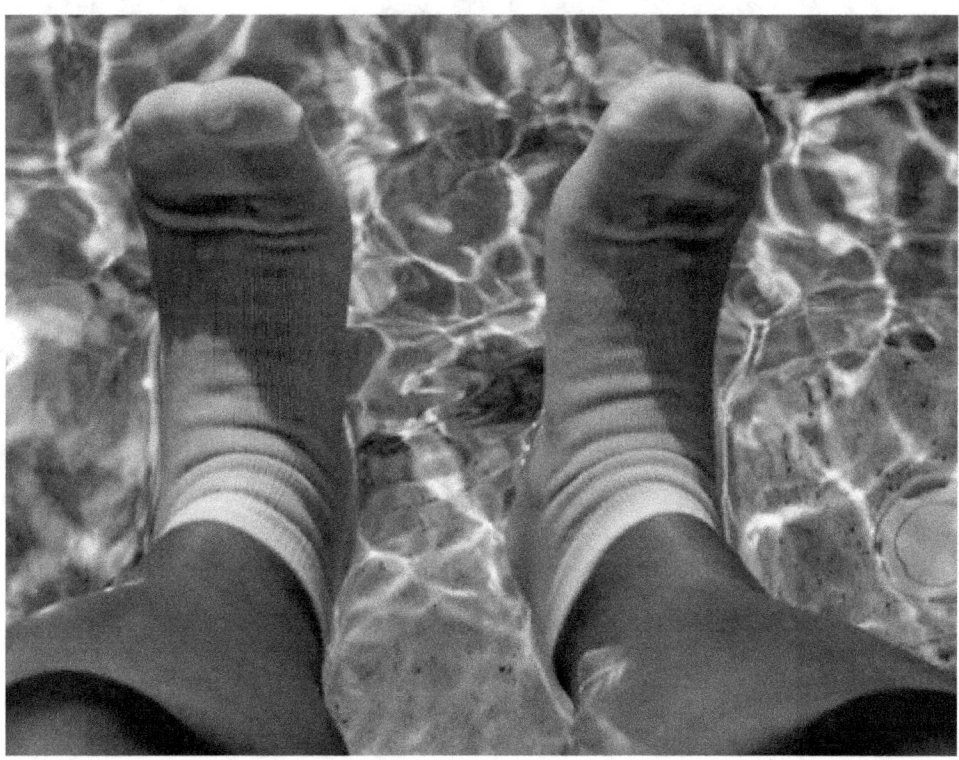

You can do this warm-up sitting in a chair before you enter the pool, or you may prefer to sit on the edge of the pool. Slowly point your toes towards you as far as you comfortably can, hold, and release. Do this exercise for a total of 8 repetitions.

Fee the stretch from each toe as your attempt to bring each toe towards you and then release it. Bring your mind and awareness to the stretch in each toes, and then to the stretch in your Achilles heel and lower calf muscle. Do not strain through this stretch.

Focus on pushing your heels away from your body. Feel the extra stretch in your calves as you perform this stretch.

2. Toes and Ankles

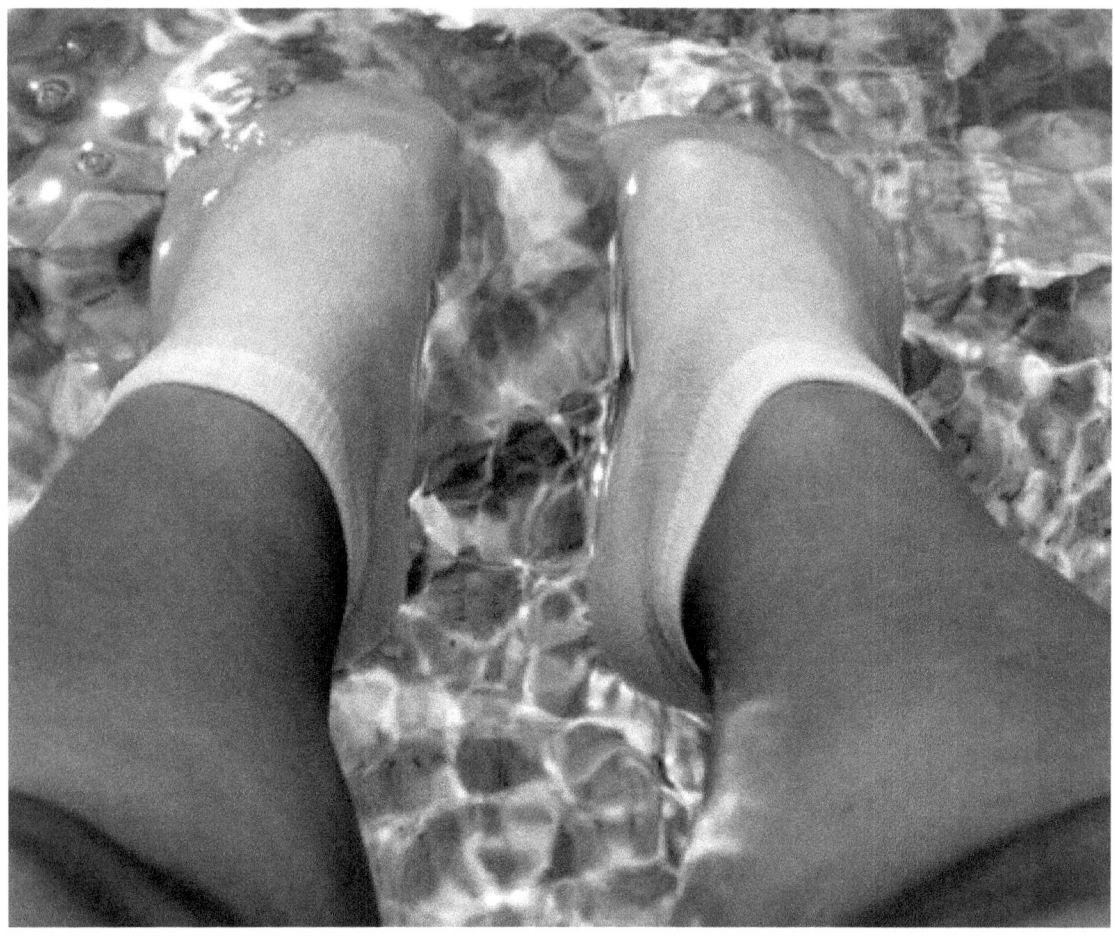

Just like in the exercise above only this time you will press your toes away from your body, hold, and then relax the stretch. Perform this stretch for eight repetitions.

Bring your focus to each of the toes and do not crunch them or fold them over one another. Allow each of the toes to enjoy and feel the stretch individually.

You will also be feeling a stretch in the front part of your leg, this is the anterior tibialis. When this muscle is not properly warmed up and stretched, many people suffer from Shin splints.

Do not over stretch this muscle, just continue pressing the toes away from you body, holding the stretch for a few seconds, and then releasing the stretch. The front of your leg should begin to feel warm.

3. Toes and Ankles

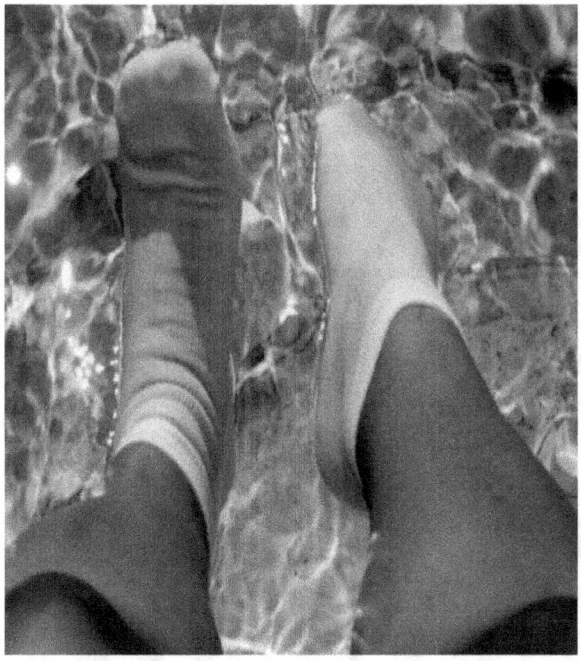 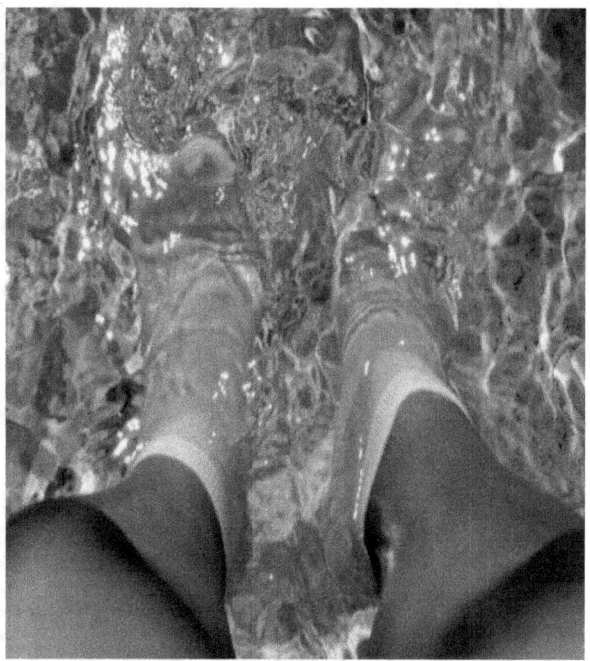

Just like in the two exercises above only this time you will press your right toes away from your body while you bring your left toes toward you body, hold for a few seconds, and then relax the stretch. Now, bring your right towed toward your body and press your left toes away from your body at the same time. Continue to alternate between your two feet in this way for a total of eight repetitions.

Bring your focus to each of the toes and do not crunch them or fold them over one another. Allow each of the toes to enjoy and feel the stretch individually.

You will also be feeling a stretch in the front part of one of your legs and a stretch on the back part of the other leg.

Do not over stretch your legs, feet, or toes, just continue alternating between pressing the toes away from you body and then towards your body, holding the stretch for a few seconds in between, and then releasing the stretch.

If you are sitting poolside, you can perform this exercise either outside of the water, or inside of the warm. The choice is up to you.

4. Toes and Ankles

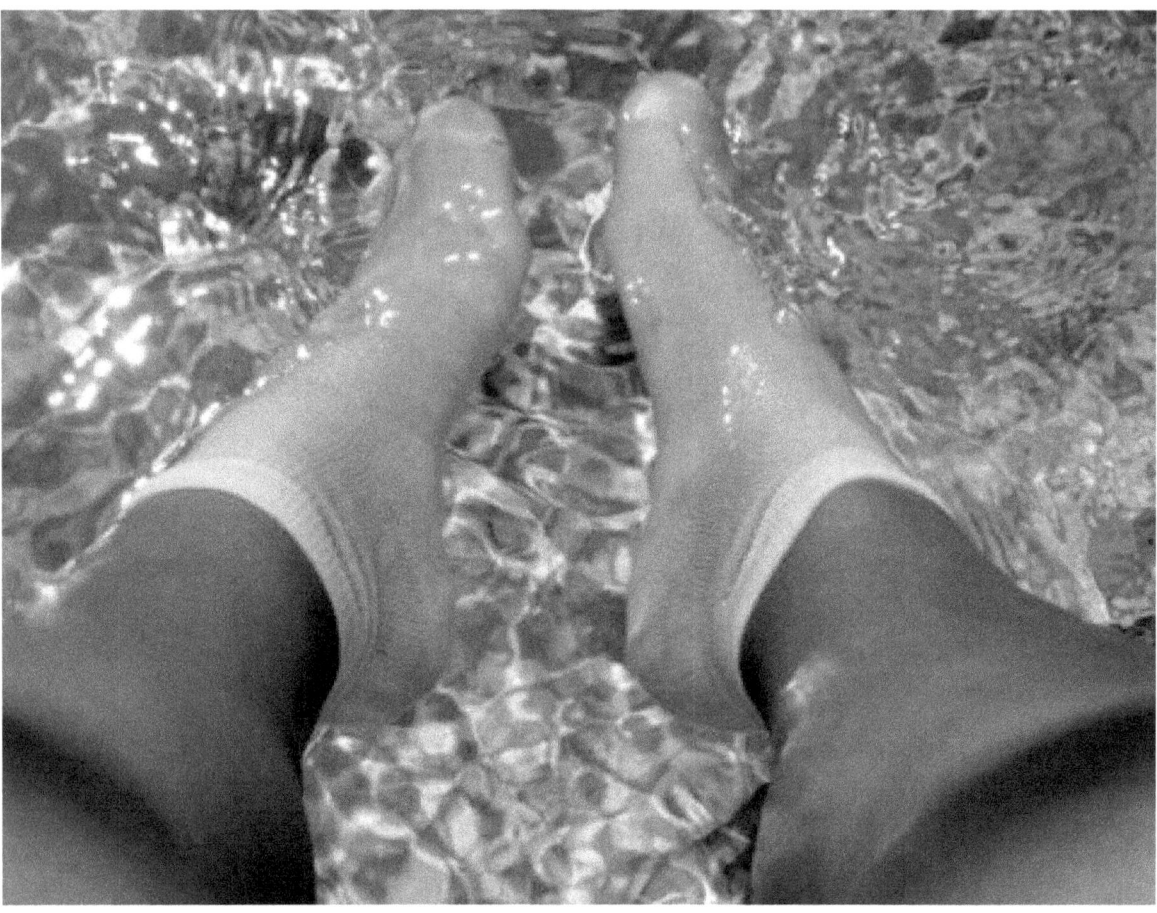

In the exercise above you will press the soles of your feet towards each other, hold for a few seconds, and then relax the stretch. Perform this stretch for eight repetitions.

Now, press the soles of your feet away from each other. Repeat for a total of eight repetitions.

Bring your focus to each of the soles of your feet and do not crunch your toes or fold them over one another.

You will also be feeling a stretch in the front part of your leg, this is the anterior tibialis. When this muscle is not properly warmed up and stretched, many people suffer from Shin splints.

Do not over stretch this muscle, just continue pressing the toes away from you body, holding the stretch for a few seconds, and then releasing the stretch. The front of your leg should begin to feel warm, as well as, your ankles.

4. Toes and Ankles

Feet Swinging

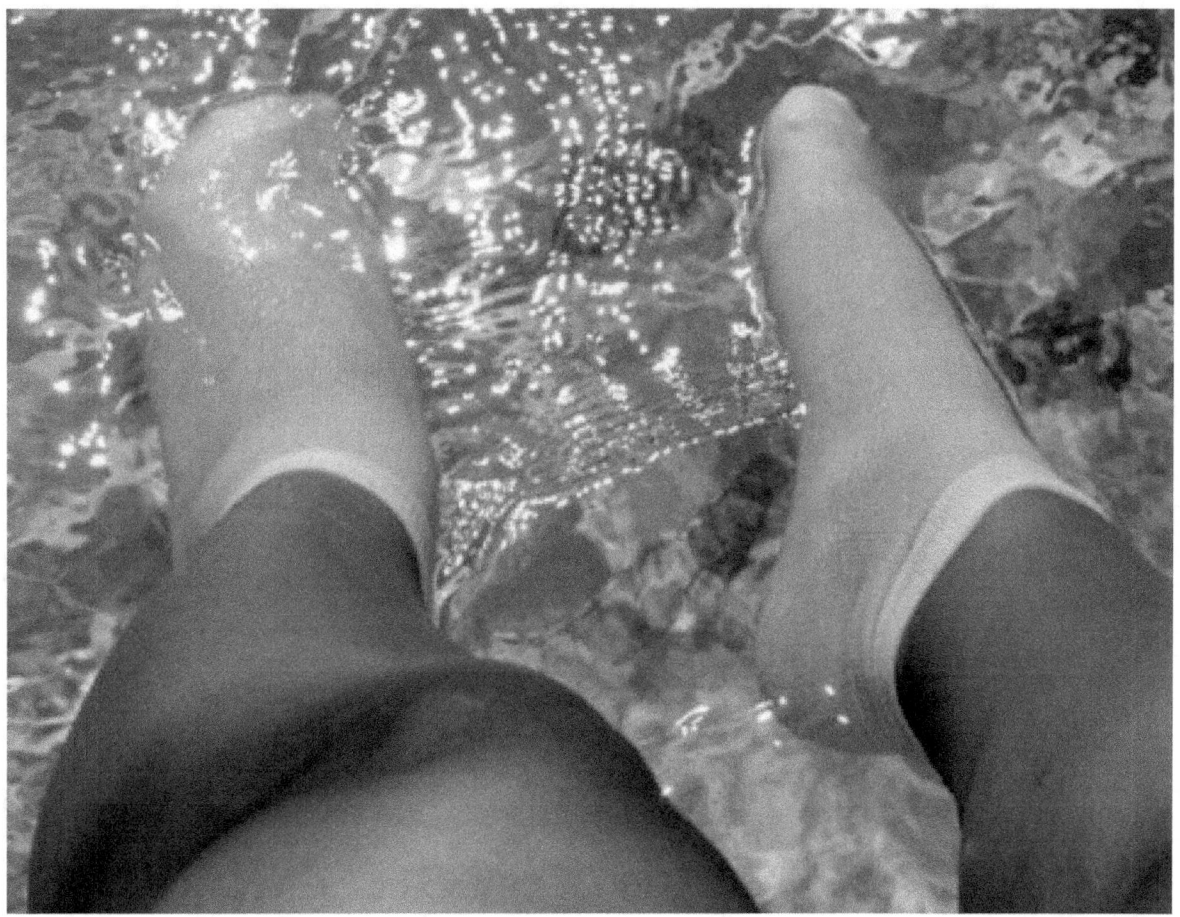

In the exercise above you will swing your feet to your right, hold for a few seconds, then swing your feet to the left, hold for a few seconds, and then relax. Perform these feet swinging exercises for eight repetitions.

Have fun with the exercise feeling the resistance of the water on your feet. Relax and enjoy.

5. Toes and Ankles

Circles

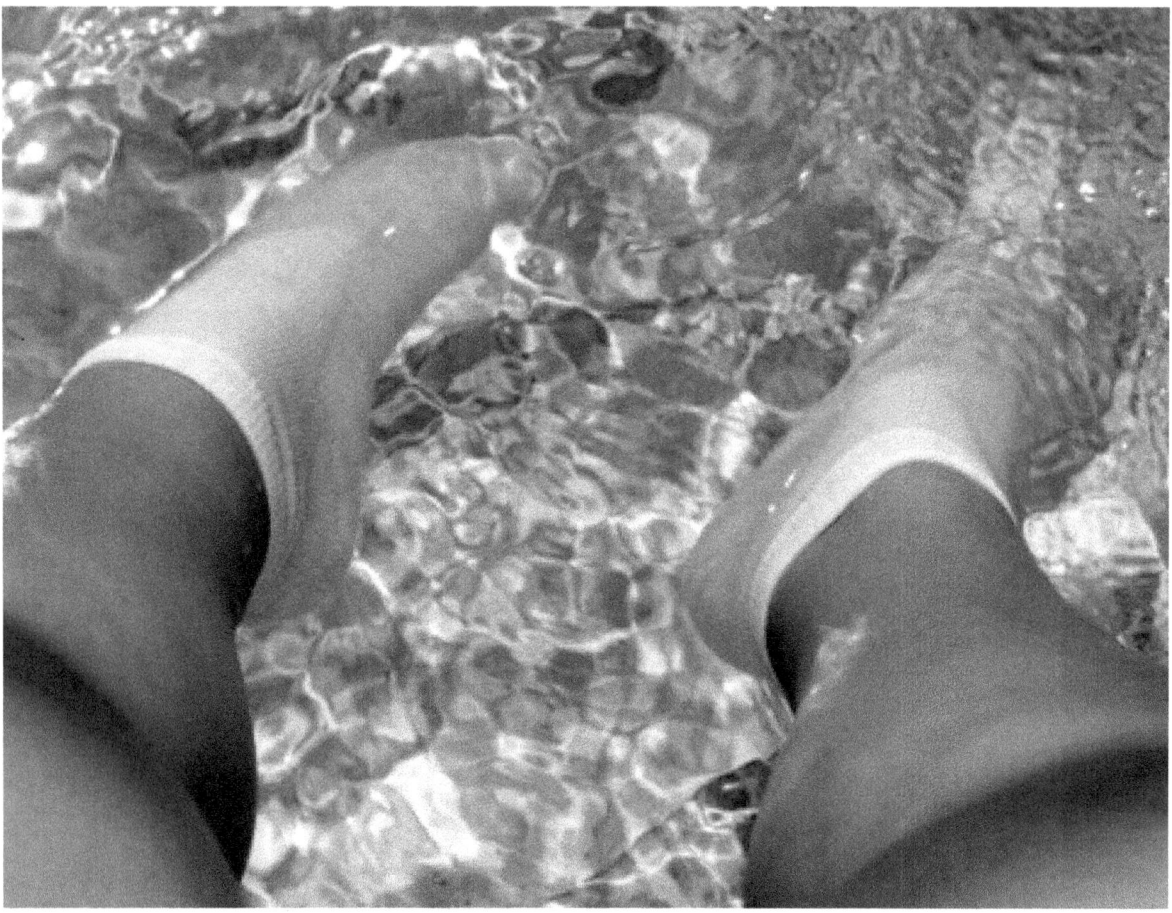

Using both feet at the same time, begin to make move your feet in a circle moving clockwise. Begin by making eight small circles and then continue to enlarge each circle until you are making eight of the largest circles you can with you feet.

Now, we will repeat the same exercise this time creating the smallest circles we can with both feet moving in a counter clockwise movement, enlarging the circles until we are able to make eight of the largest counter clockwise circle we can.

You should be able to feel a nice warmth or heat in your ankles by this time. If this exercise is painful in anyway, stop the exercise immediately and consult with you primary care physician.

Warm-ups for the Neck

     Like the warm-ups for the toes and ankles, warm-ups for the neck can be performed on land before you enter the water environment. Do not push these stretches beyond what your physical capabilities are. Stretches should not be painful. If they are, stop immediately and consult with your primary health care provider.

Neck Warm-ups

1. Neck

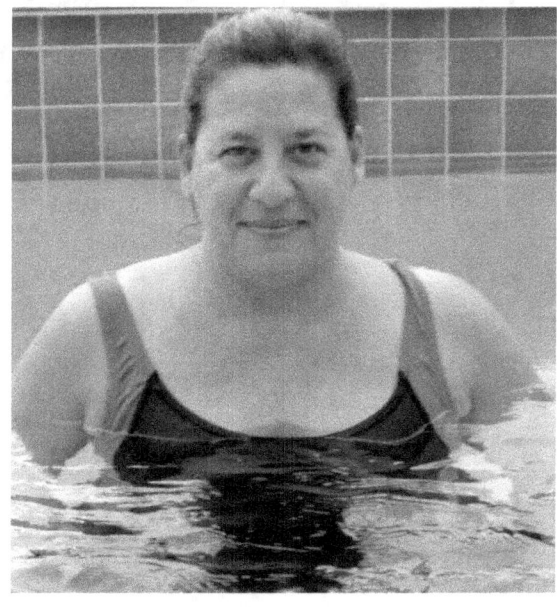 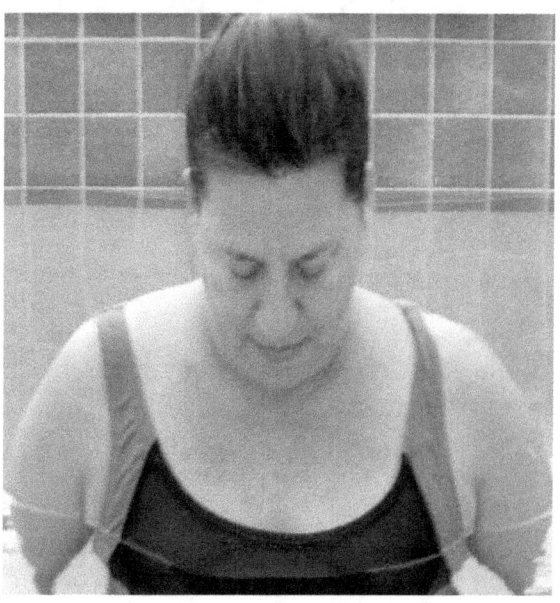

Starting Position

     The starting point for the neck exercises will begin with the head in a neutral position as is shown in the diagram above, on the left. Keep you gaze in front of you at a slight angle downward. Be sure to breathe normally.

     With your head in the starting position take a nice deep slow breath in. As you exhale, slowly allow your head to fall forward touching your chin to your chest (note: if you cannot touch your chin to your chest, this is alright, don't force the movement.)

     Now, slowly inhale and begin to return your head to the starting position. Repeat this exercise for a total of eight repetitions.

2. Neck

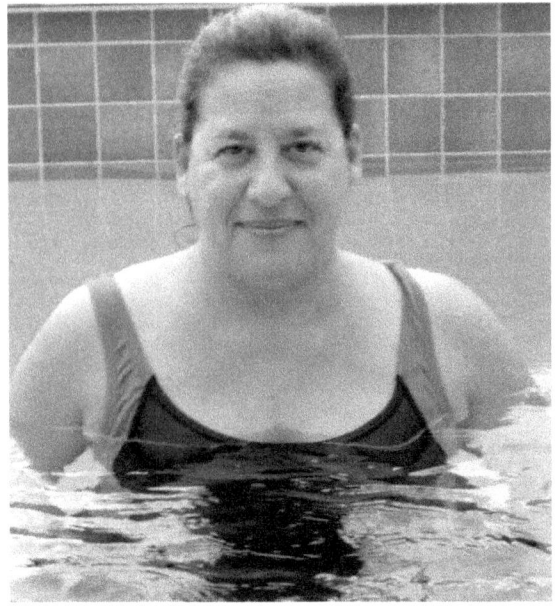 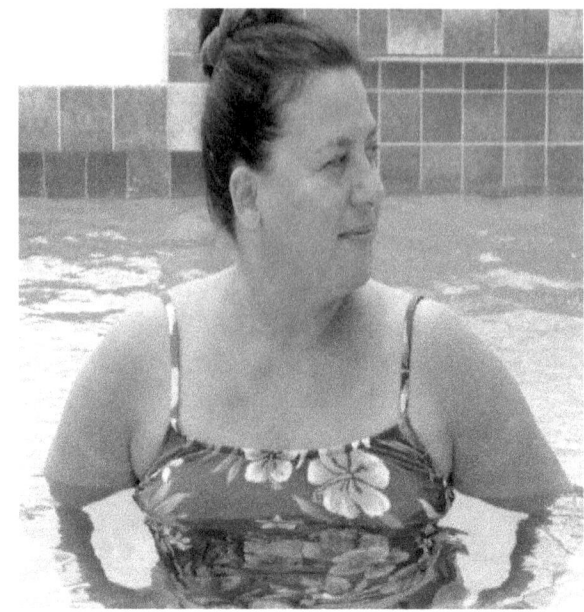

With your head in the starting position take a nice deep slow breath in. As you exhale, slowly turn your head to left aligning your chin to over your left shoulder (note: if you cannot align your chin to over your shoulder, this is alright, don't force the movement.)

Now, slowly inhale and as you exhale, begin to return your head to the starting position.

With your head in the starting position take a nice deep slow breath in. As you exhale, slowly turn your head to right aligning your chin to over your right shoulder (note: if you cannot align your chin to over your shoulder, this is alright, don't force the movement.)

Repeat this exercise for a total of eight repetitions.

3. Neck

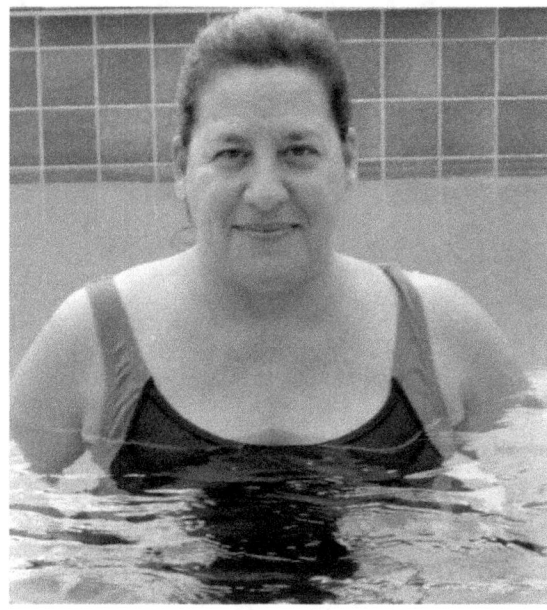 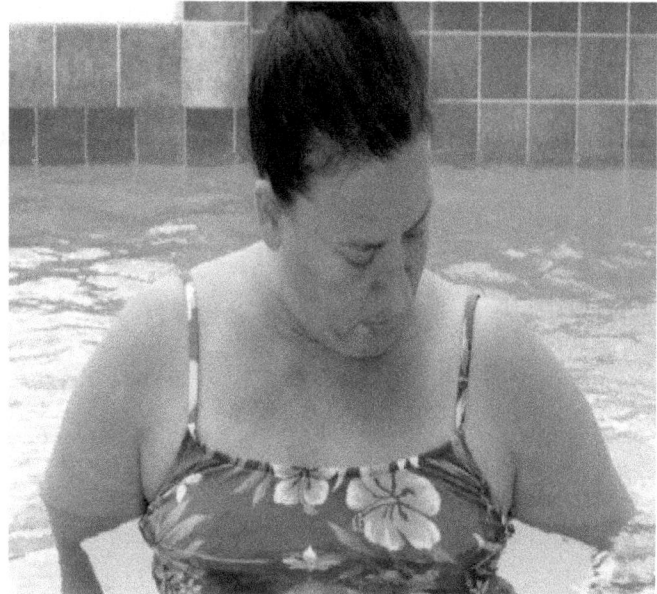

With your head in the starting position take a nice deep slow breath in. As you exhale, slowly allow your chin to drop to the left to a point that is located half way between the center of your chest and your left shoulder (note: if you cannot touch your chin to your chest, this is alright, don't force the movement.)

Now, slowly inhale and as you exhale, begin to return your head to the starting position.

With your head in the starting position take a nice deep slow breath in. As you exhale, slowly allow your chin to drop to the right to a point that is located half way between the center of your chest and your right shoulder (note: if you cannot touch your chin to your chest, this is alright, don't force the movement.)

Repeat this exercise for a total of eight repetitions.

4. Neck

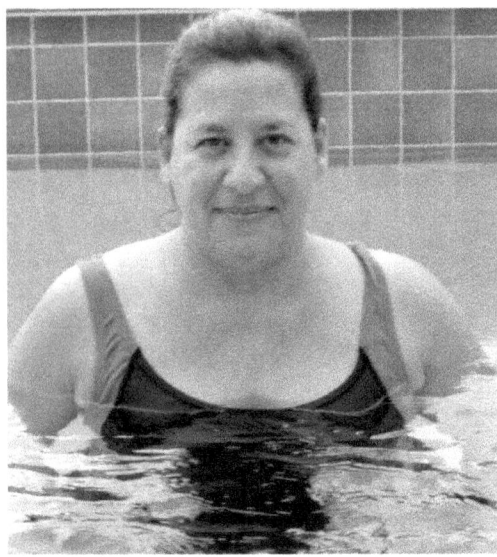 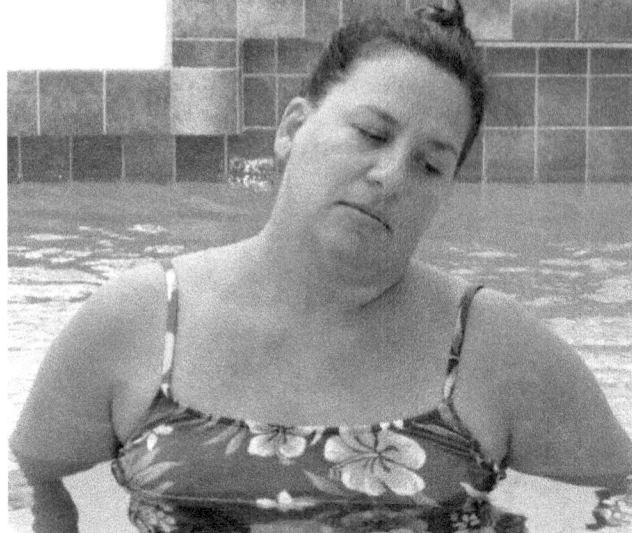

With your head in the starting position take a nice deep slow breath in. As you exhale, slowly allow your left ear to drop to your left shoulder (note: if you cannot touch your ear to your shoulder, this is alright, don't force the movement.)

Now, slowly inhale and as you exhale, begin to return your head to the starting position.

With your head in the starting position take a nice deep slow breath in. As you exhale, slowly allow your right ear to drop to your right shoulder (note: if you cannot touch your ear to your shoulder, this is alright, don't force the movement.)

Repeat this exercise for a total of eight repetitions.

5. Neck

Head Rolls

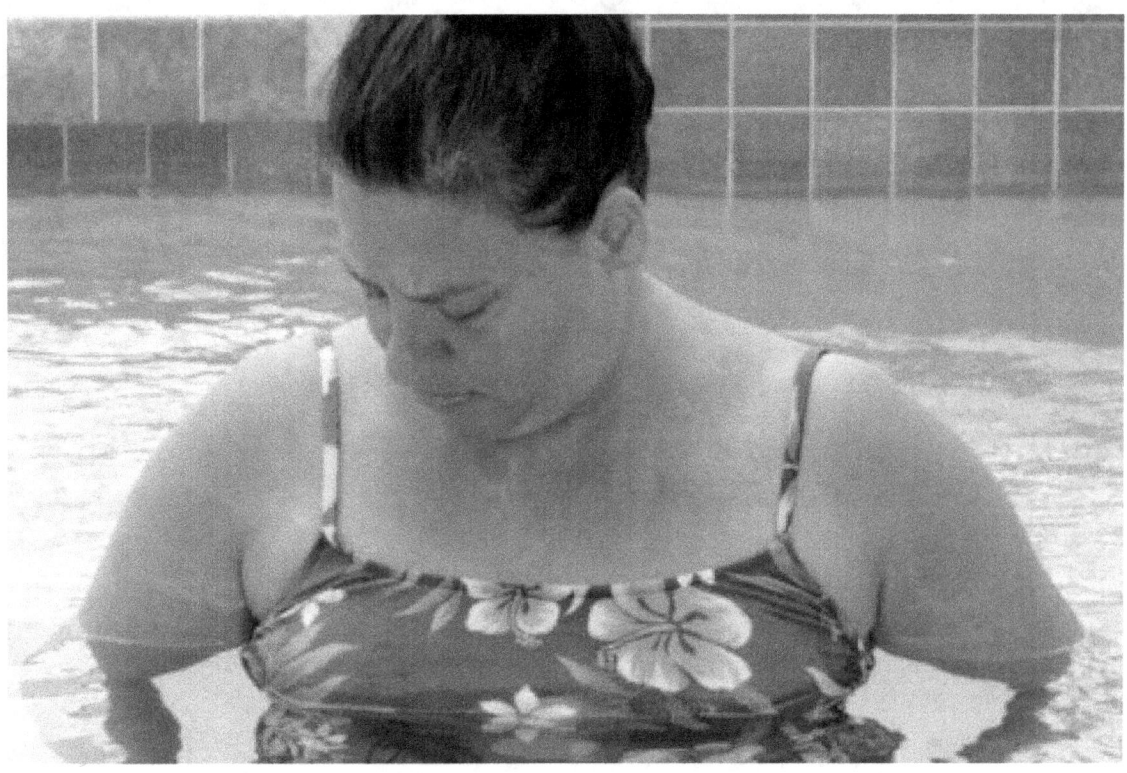

For this exercise you will imagine that your nose is like the hands of wall clock. The numbers of the wall clock are right in front of your face.

To begin, you will take a nice deep slow breath in and as you slowly exhale you will begin with your nose in the twelve o'clock position. Moving clockwise outline the numbers of the clock from 3, to 6, to 9, and ending back at the top at the number 12 position.

Repeat for eight repetitions.

Now, repeat the above exercise, this time moving counter clockwise beginning at the 12 position moving down to the 9, 6, 3, and back to the top 12 position.

Repeat for eight repetitions.

1. Shoulders

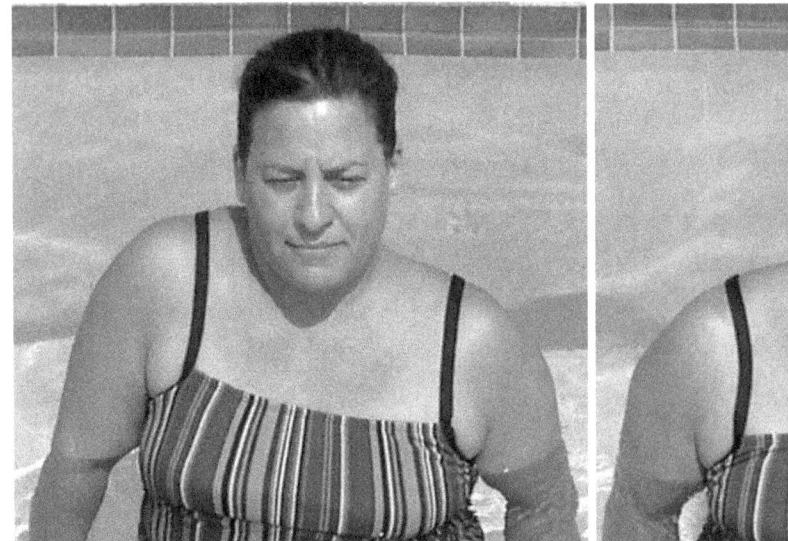 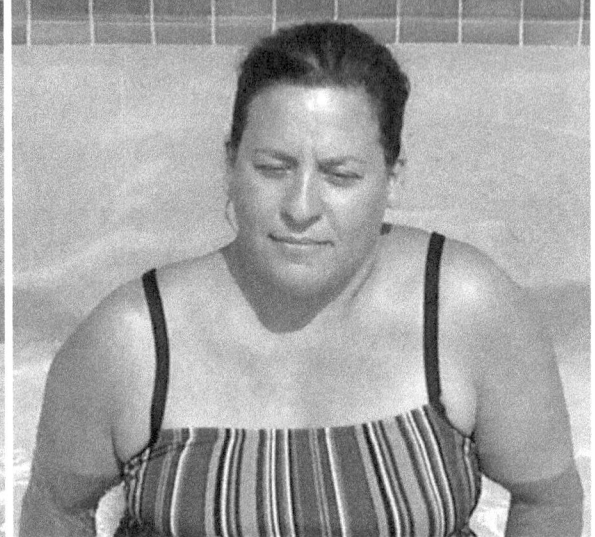

Begin by planting both feet flat on the bottom of the pool. Bend your knees slightly and arms down at your sides. Now, standing perfectly straight, inhale and bring your right shoulder up to your right ear and hold. As you exhale release the shoulder back down to starting position. Remember-do NOT bring your ear down to meet the shoulder. This is very important. Repeat for a total of 8 repetitions.

Now, inhale and bring your left shoulder up to your left ear and hold. As you exhale, relax and return to the starting position. Repeat for a total of 8 repetitions.

Alternating Shoulders: Inhale and bring your right shoulder up to your right ear and hold. Exhale and relax the shoulder back to the starting position. Inhale and bring your left shoulder up to your left ear and hold. Exhale and relax the shoulder back to the starting position. Repeat for a total of 16 repetitions. Do NOT bring ears to shoulders.

2. Shoulders – Shrugs

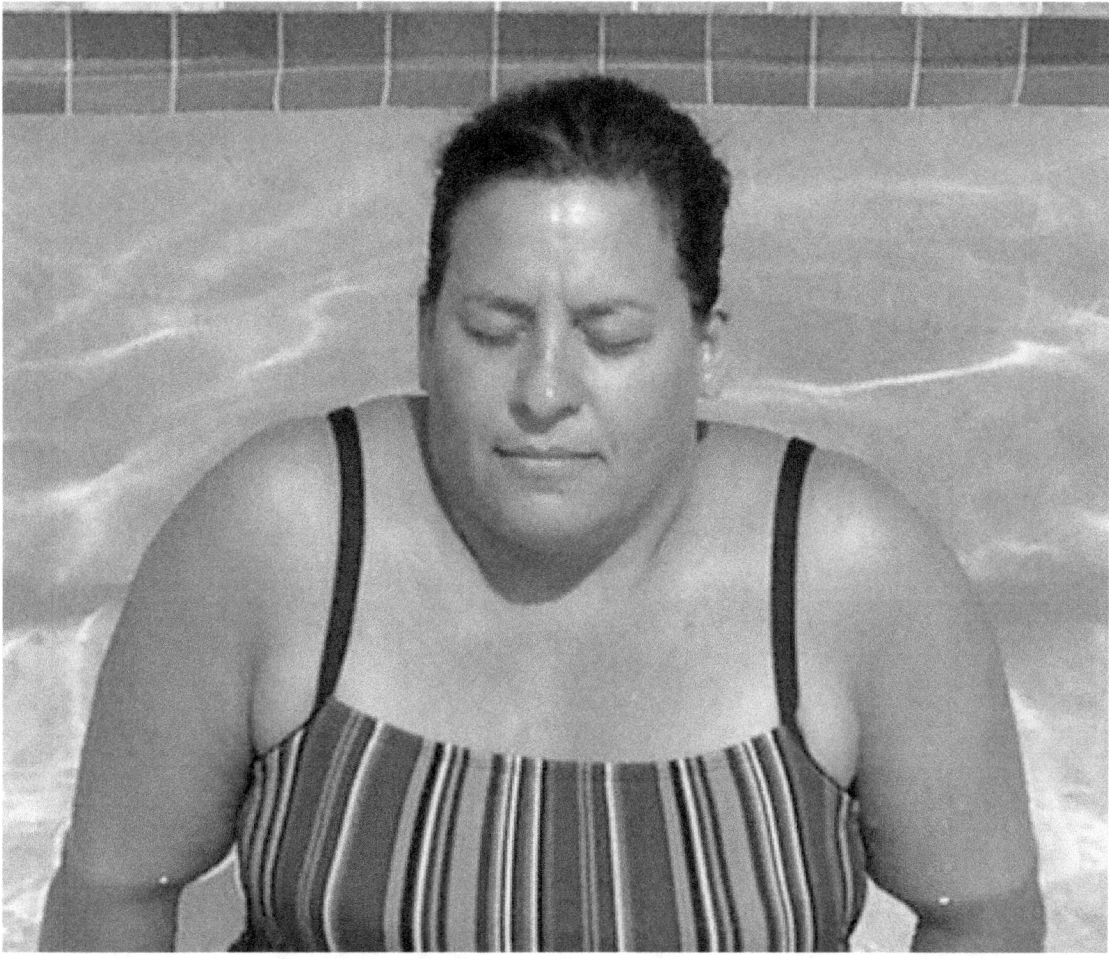

    Inhale and bring both of your shoulders up to your ears and hold for a few seconds. As you exhale, allow both shoulders to relax and return to the starting position. Continue for a total of 16 repetitions.

This is a great exercise to do through out the day to reduce stress.

3. Shoulders – Circles

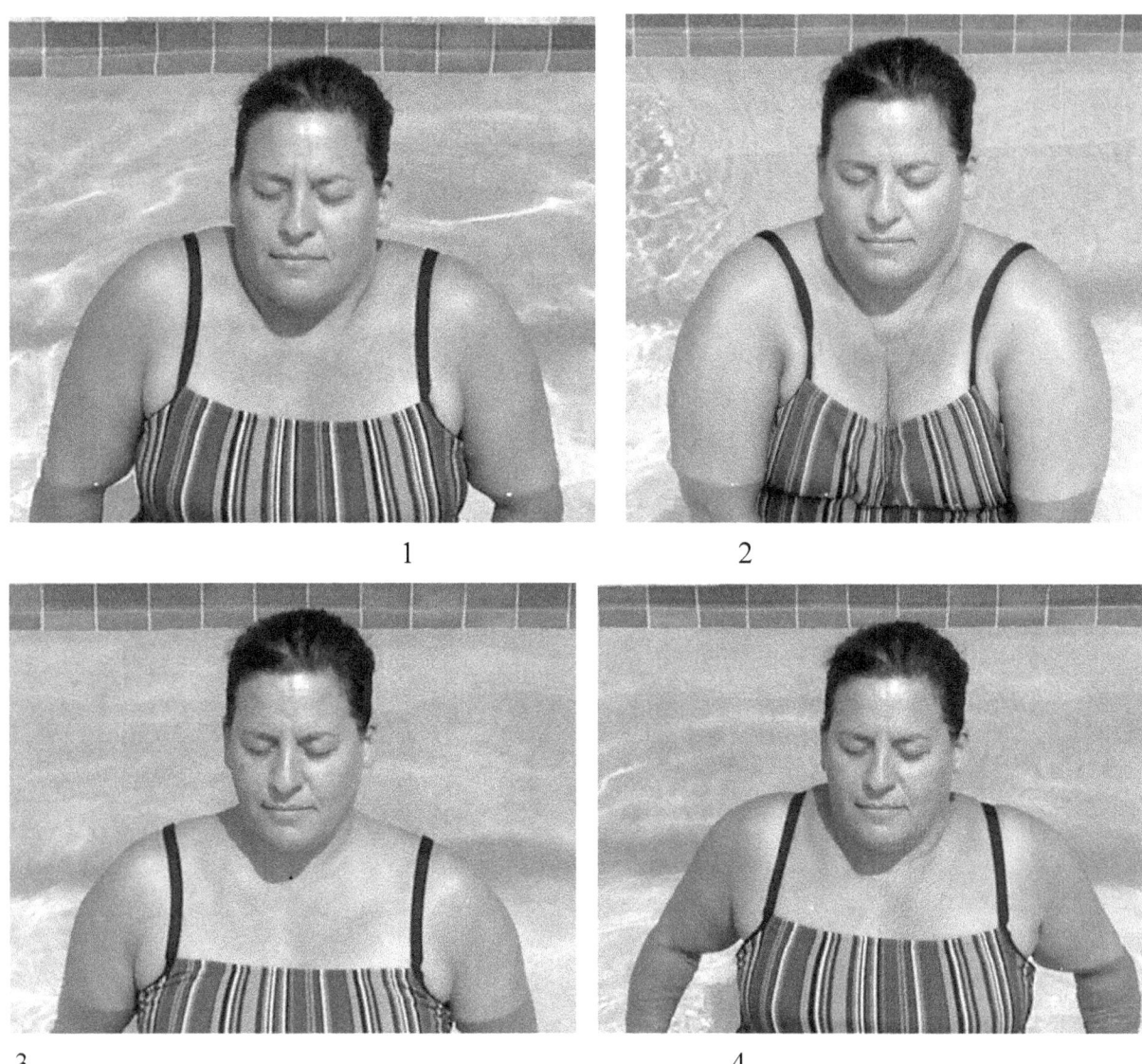

1

2

3

4

Inhale and bring both shoulders up to your ears (1) and as you exhale allow the shoulders to push forward (2), then down (3), then back behind you (4) forming a circle. As you inhale again pull the shoulders back up to your ears and repeat the circle of exhaling and allowing the shoulders to drop to the front, down to the sides and to the back before returning up to the ears again. Repeat for a total of 8 repetitions.

When finished, repeat this exercise, this time inhaling and bringing the ears up to the shoulders and as you exhale, allowing the shoulders to drop towards the back, down to the sides, up to the front and back up to the ears in the next inhalation. (4-3-2-1). Repeat for a total of 8 repetitions.

Warm-up for the Wrists

1. Wrists

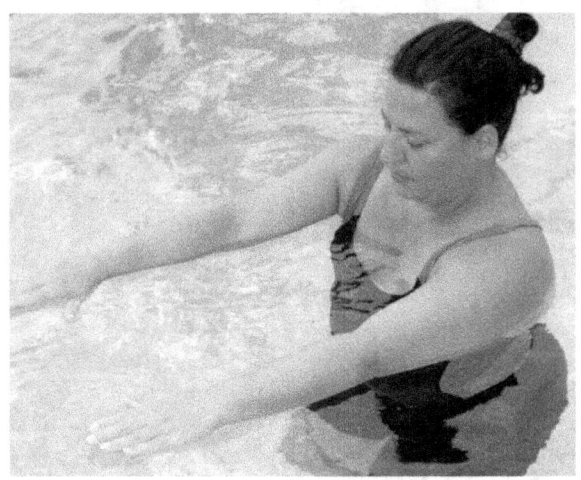 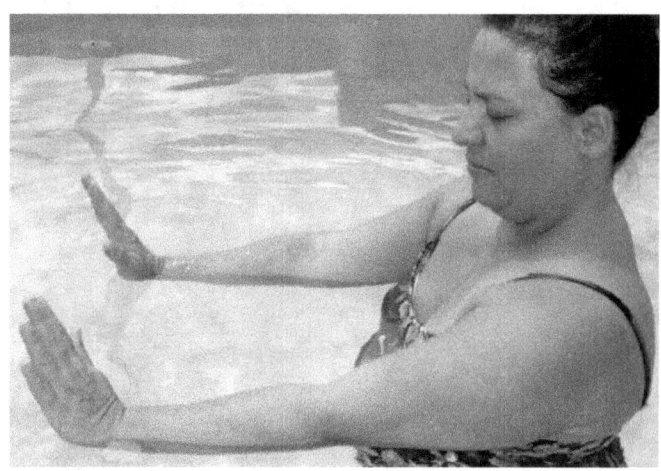

Starting Position:

Begin the following exercises in the starting position as shown in the picture above on the left. To begin, make sure that both of your feet are planted firmly on the bottom of the pool.

Bend your knees and be sure that they are shoulder width apart. Extend both of your arms straight out in front of your body with fingers pointing away from your body. This is the starting position.

To do the exercise:

Take a nice slow, deep breath and at the same time, lift the fingers of both of your hands towards you while keeping the heel of your hand pushing away from your body, hold the stretch for a few seconds.

As you slowly exhale, lower your fingers back to the starting position as shown in the picture above, on the left.

Repeat for a total of eight repetitions.

2. Wrists

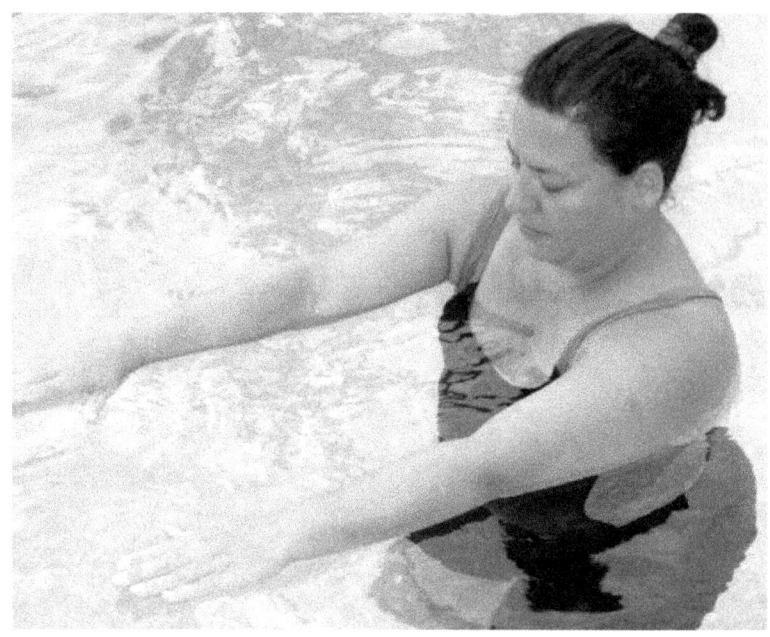

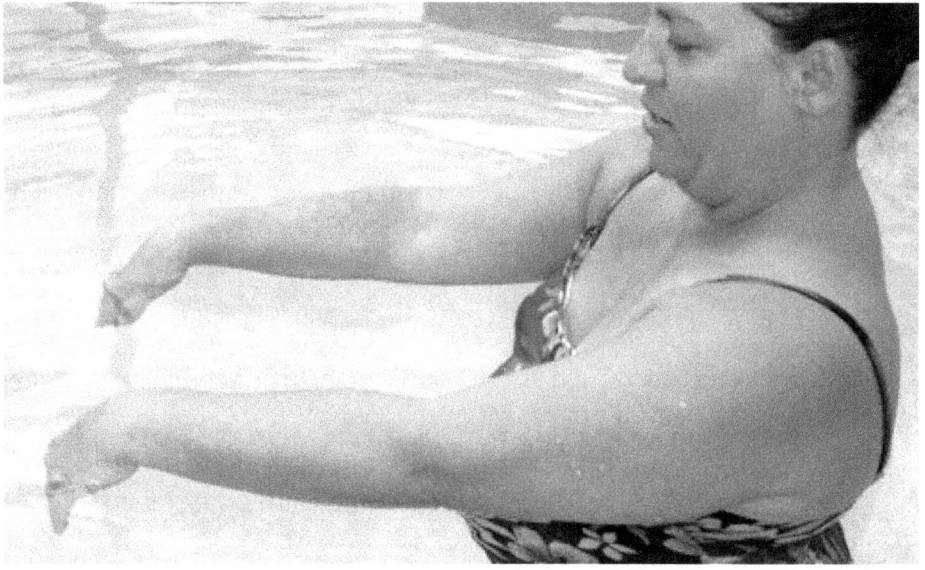

Extend both of your arms straight out in front of your body. Do not lock your elbows. If this is uncomfortable, just relax your arms and do the best that you can.

Take a nice slow, deep breath and at the same time, point the fingers of both of your hands down towards the bottom of the pool, while keeping you arms extended away from your body, hold the stretch for a few seconds.

As you slowly exhale, raise your fingers back to the starting position as shown in the picture above, on the left. Repeat for a total of eight repetitions.

3. Wrists

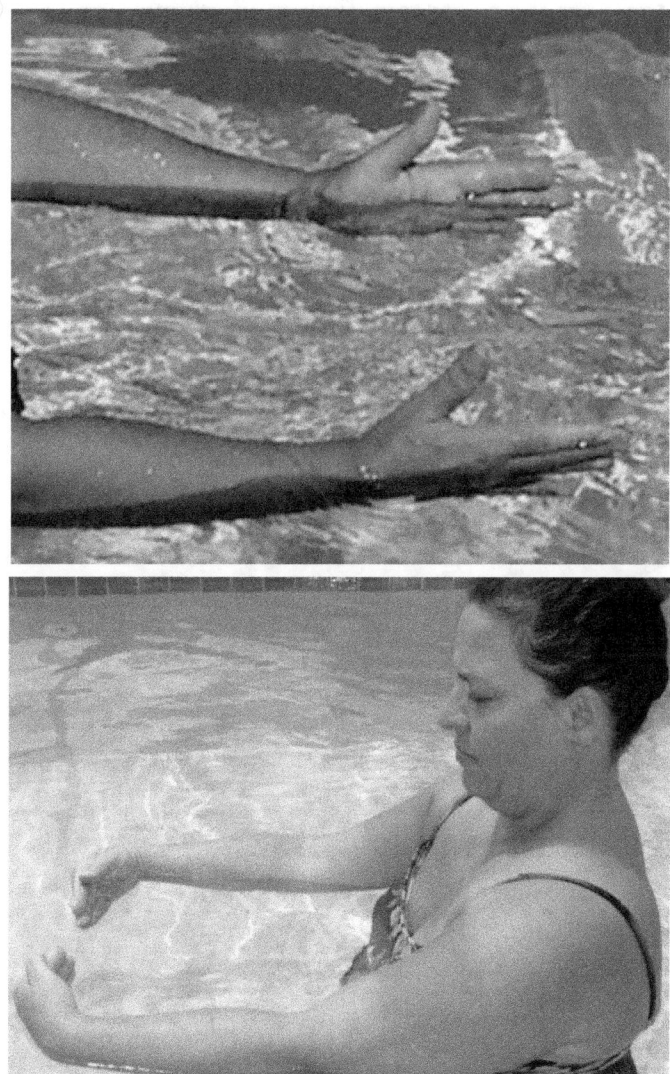

Extend both of your arms straight out in front of your body. Do not lock your elbows. If this is uncomfortable, just relax your arms and do the best that you can.

Take a nice slow, deep breath and at the same time, point the fingers of both of your hands towards each other while keeping your arms extended in front of your body, hold the stretch for a few seconds.

As you slowly exhale, lower your fingers back to the starting position. Repeat for a total of eight repetitions.

4. Wrists

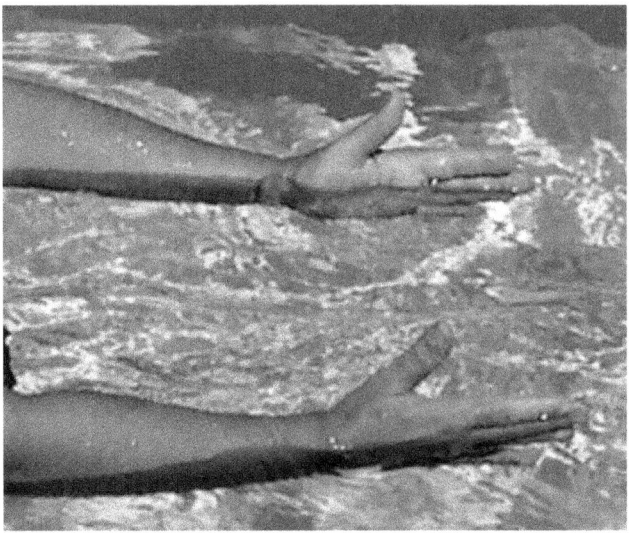

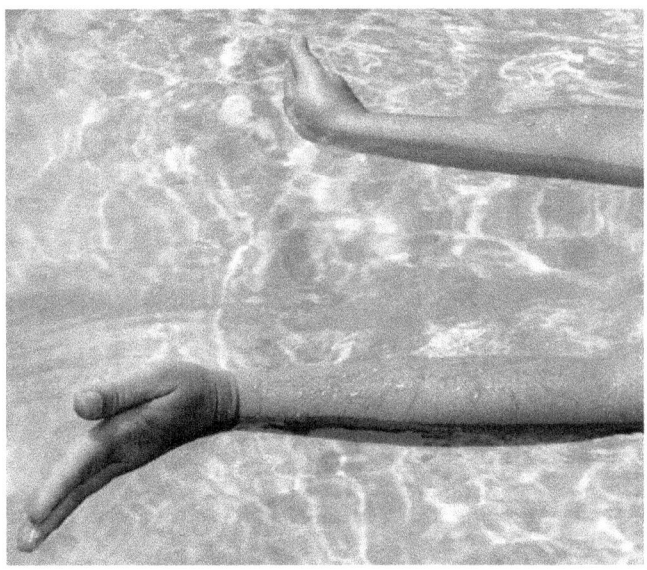

Extend both of your arms straight out in front of your body. Do not lock your elbows. If this is uncomfortable, just relax your arms and do the best that you can.

Take a nice slow, deep breath and at the same time, point the fingers of both of your hands away from each other while keeping your arms extended straight in front of your body, hold the stretch for a few seconds.

As you slowly exhale, return your fingers back to the starting position. Repeat for a total of eight repetitions.

5. Wrists

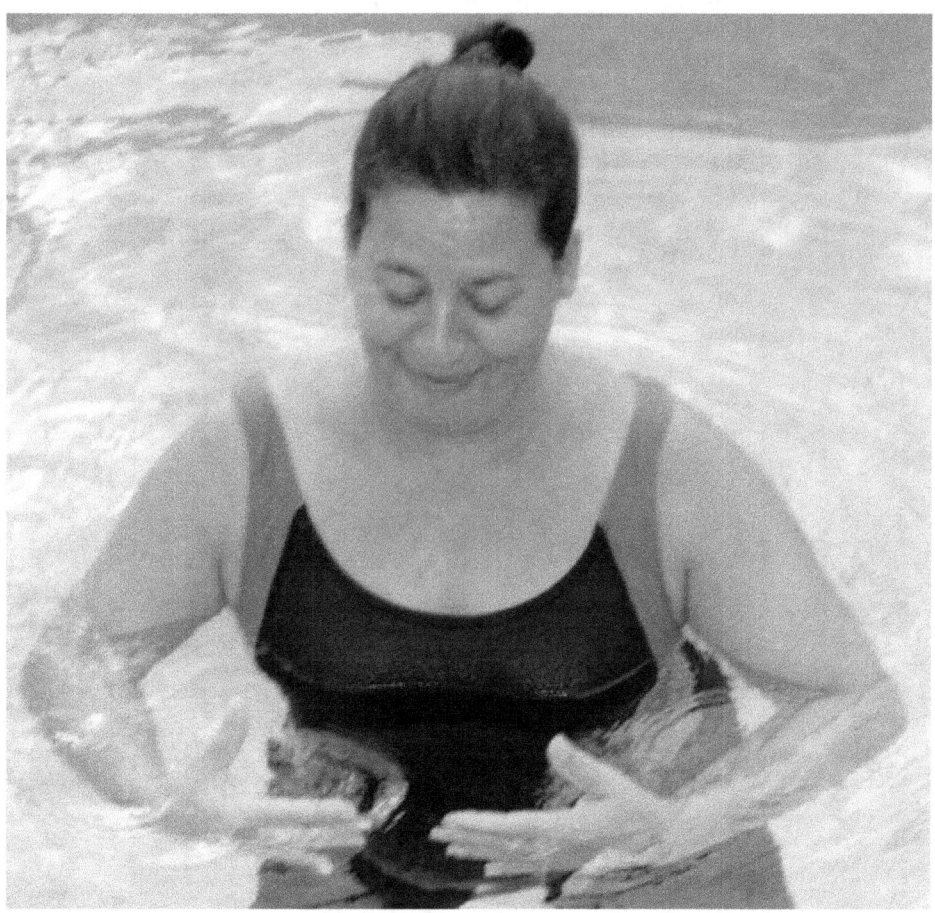

Circles

Extend both of your arms straight out in front of your body. Do not lock your elbows. If this is uncomfortable, just relax your arms and do the best that you can.

Begin with your fingers facing each other as shown in the picture above. Make outward circles with your wrists. (The right hand will be making clockwise circles and the left hand will be making counter clockwise circles at the same time.) Do for eight repetitions.

Then, reverse the direction. The right hand will then be making counter clockwise circles and the left hand will be making clockwise circles. Do for eight repetitions.

You should feel nice warmth in your wrists with this exercise. It is also very invigorating after a day of typing or craft work.

6. Wrist and Forearm

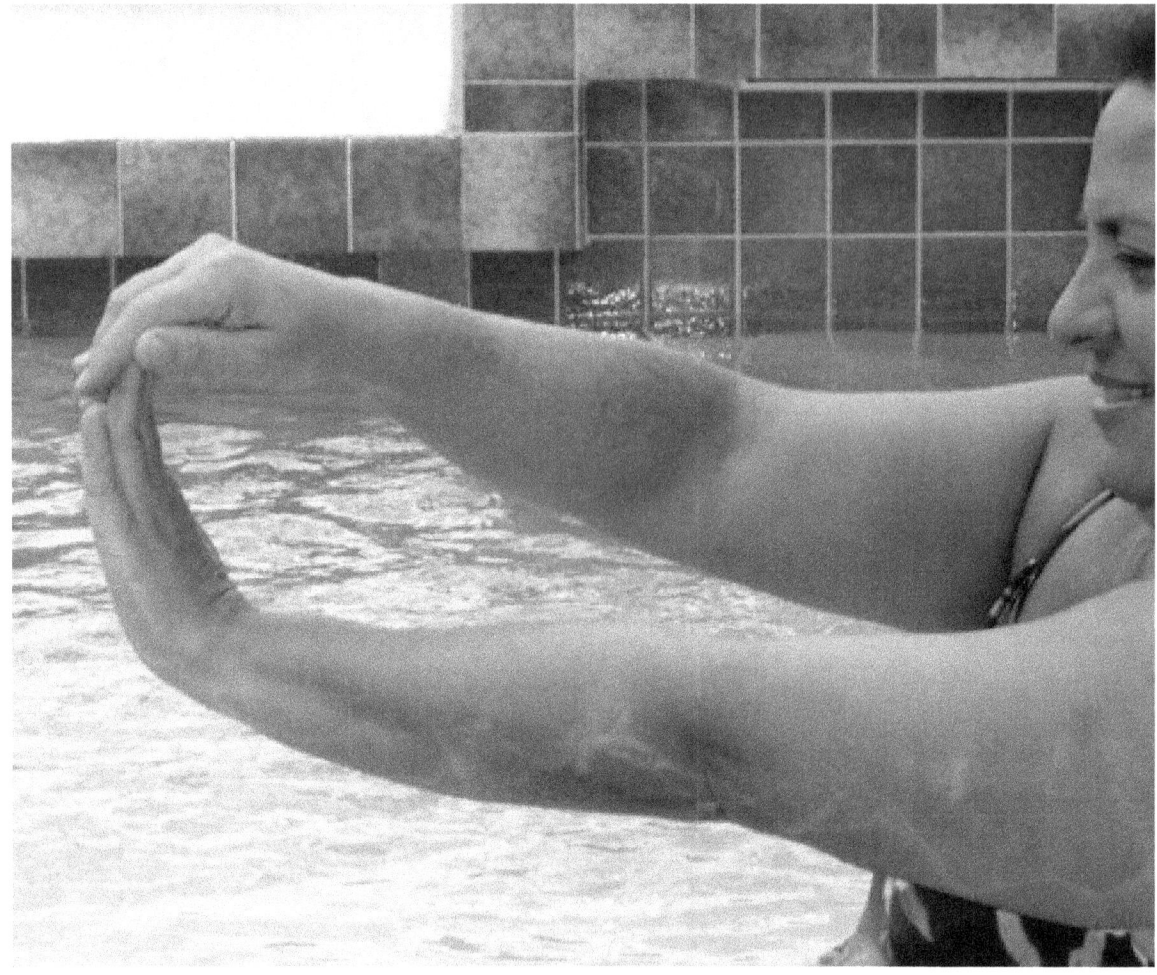

Extend your left arm straight out from the front of your body with your fingers pointed upward.

Extend your right arm straight out from the front of your body on top of your left arm and gently grab on to the fingers of your left hand.

Now, take a nice slow deep breath in. As you exhale, gently apply pressure to the fingers of the left hand pressing them toward the front of your body; hold the stretch for a few seconds, then release.

Repeat the exercise for a total of eight repetitions. Do not over stretch.

7. Wrist and Forearm

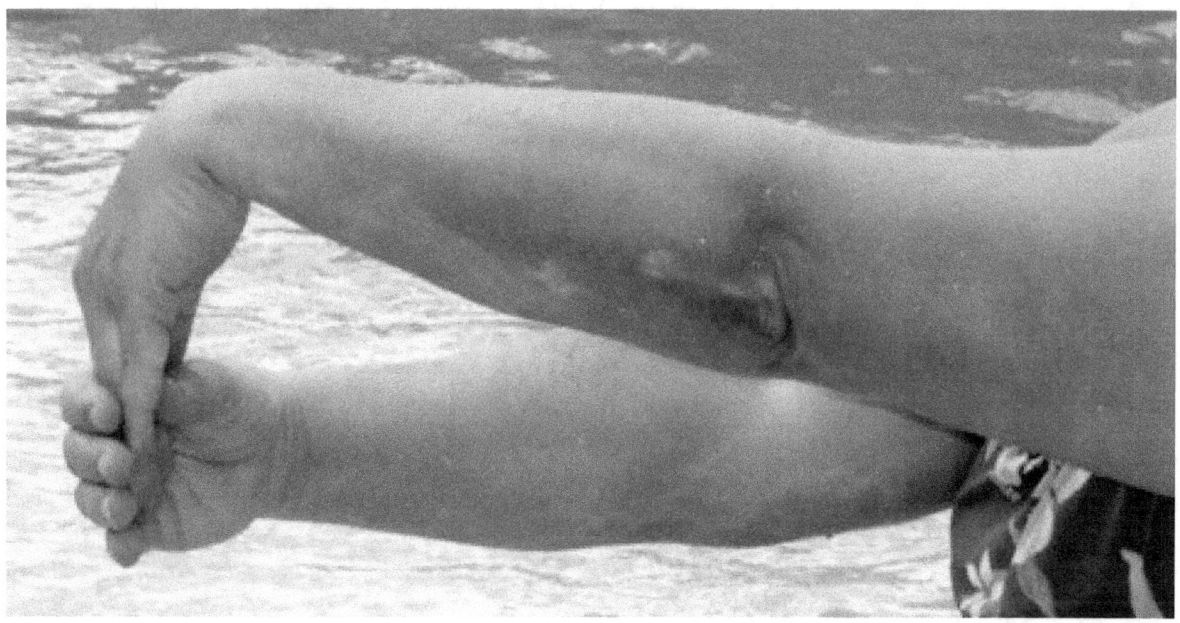

Extend your left arm straight out from the front of your body with your fingers pointed down towards the bottom of the pool.

Extend your right arm straight out from the front of your body on the bottom of your left arm and gently grab on to the fingers of your left hand.

Now, take a nice slow deep breath in. As you exhale, gently apply pressure to the fingers of the left hand pressing them toward the front of your body; hold the stretch for a few seconds, then release.

Repeat the exercise for a total of eight repetitions.

Do not over stretch.

Making a fist

You can put together the above wrist exercises in a unique way. Try performing the above exercises with your hands closed in a fist. This will add a slight additional stretch to the muscles in the wrists and forearm.

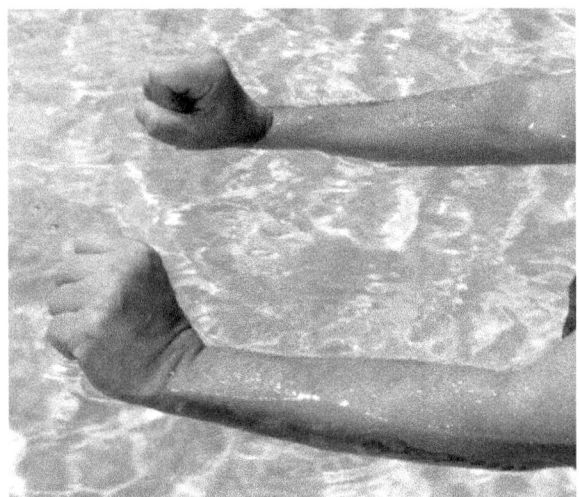 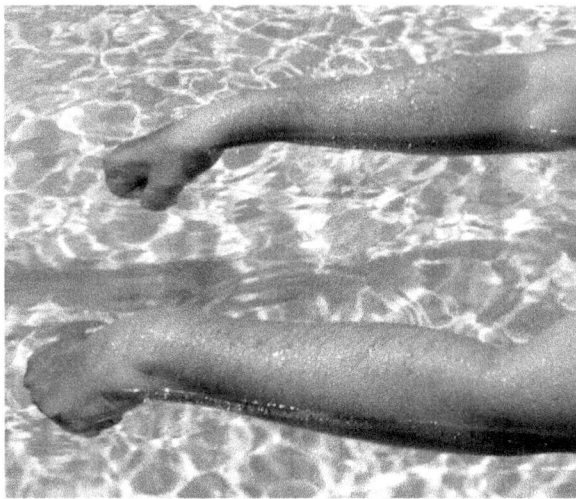

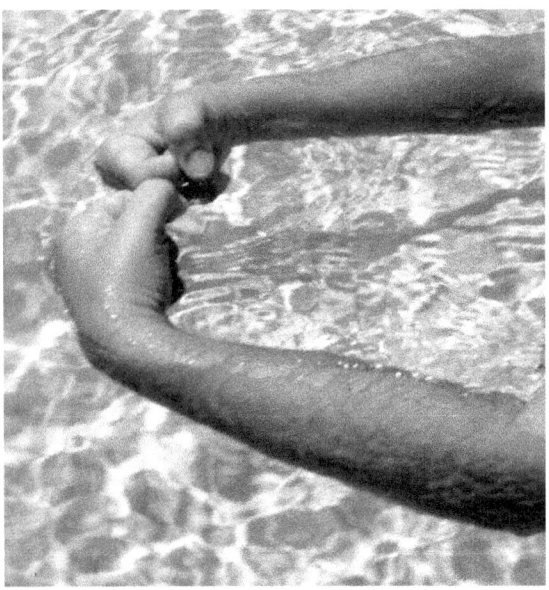 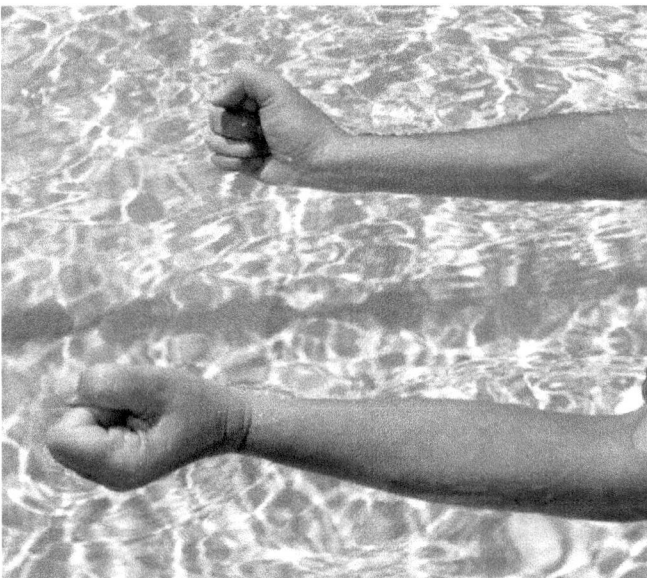

Warm ups for the Arms

1. Arms

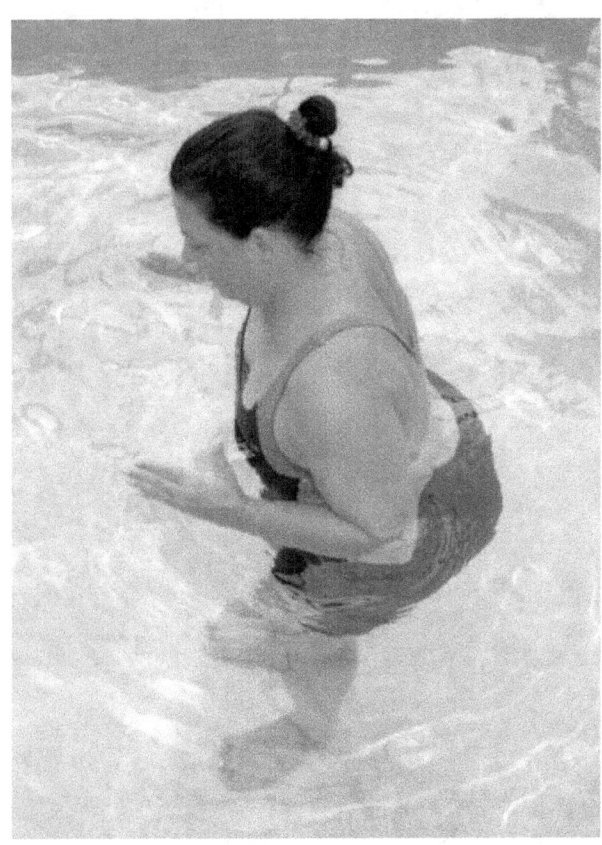 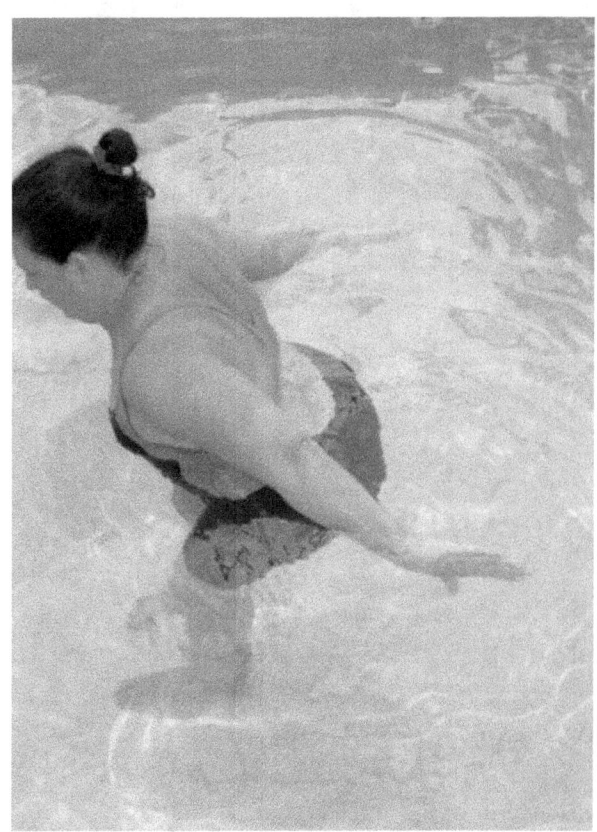

To Do:

Plant both of your feet flat on the bottom of the pool at shoulder width apart. There should be approximately 6" to 8" of space between your feet.

Bend your knees and find the balance in your body. Bend your elbows and bring your hands up towards you shoulders as shown in the picture above on the left. Your thumbs should be pointing towards your shoulders.

Now, slowly straighten your arms, bringing them through the water to as far back as you comfortably can, hold, and release back to starting point. Notice that the thumbs are now pointing towards the bottom of the pool. Do a total of eight repetitions.

2. Arms

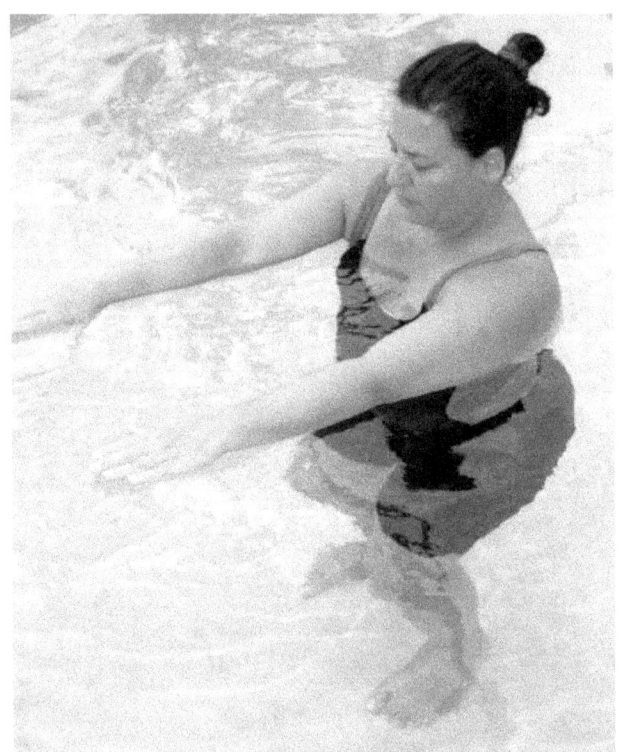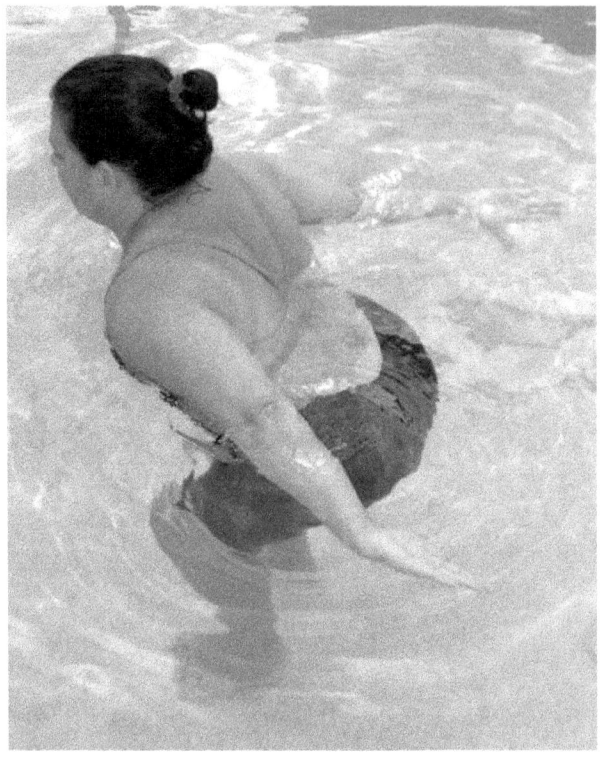

To Do:

Plant both feet flat on the bottom of the pool at shoulder width apart. Be sure that there is approximately 6" to 8" of space between your feet. Bend your knees and find the balance point for your body.

Place your arms straight out in front of your body as shown in the picture above on the left. The thumbs of each hand are facing in towards each other.

Now, slowly bring your arms down into the water, and sweep them back as far as you comfortably can, hold, and release back to starting point. Do a total of eight repetitions.

5. Arms and Shoulders

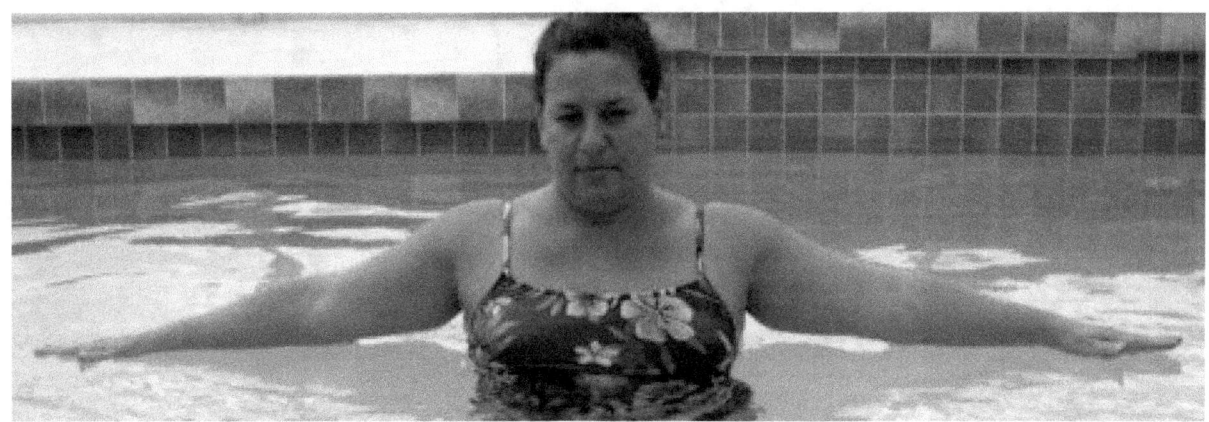

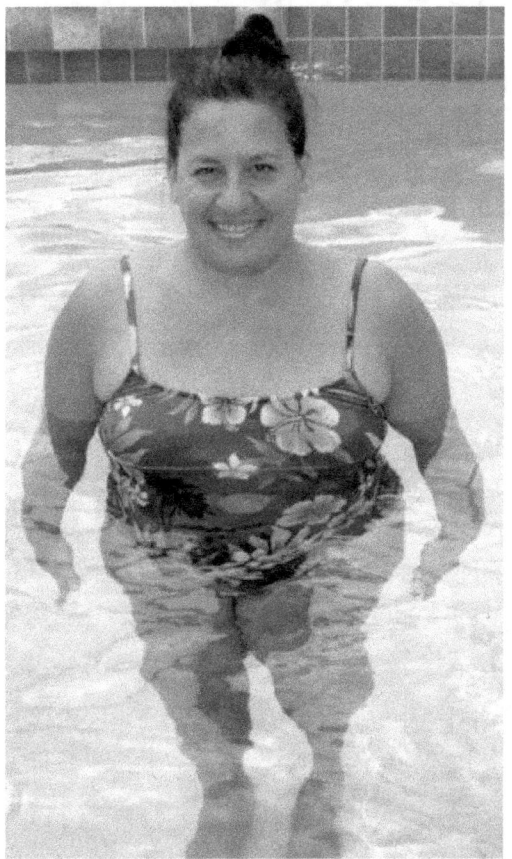

To Do:

Place your straight out from your sides as shown in the picture above. Now, slowly bring both of your arms down into the water towards your side, hold, and release back to starting point. Do a total of eight repetitions.

6. Arms and Shoulders

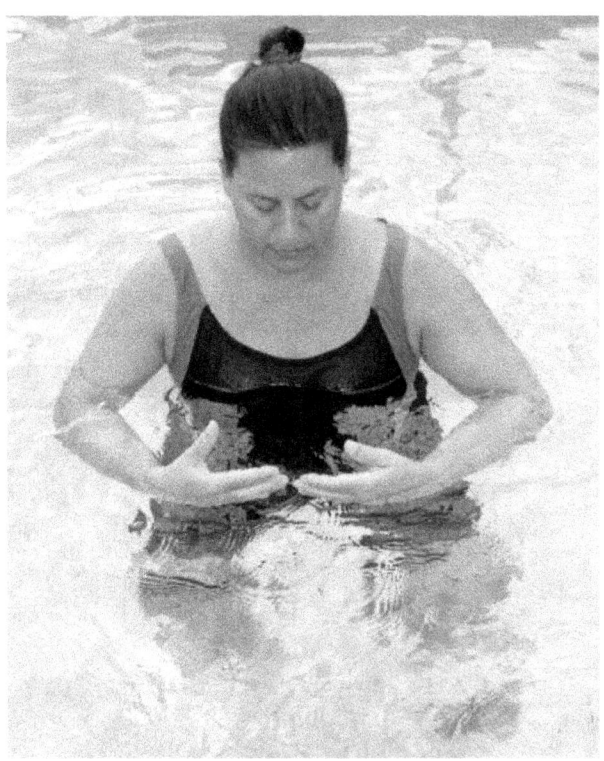

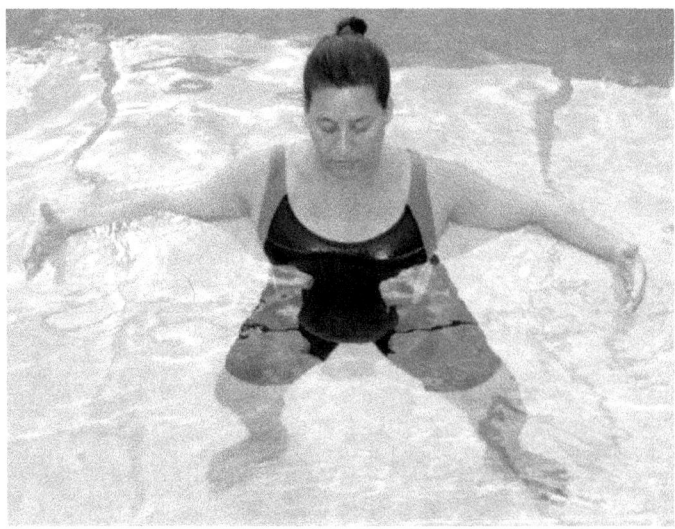

To Do:

Bend your knees and bring your hands in front of your body as shown in the picture above. Now, slowly pull your elbows backwards opening your chest, hold, and release back to starting point. Do a total of eight repetitions.

7. Arms and Shoulders

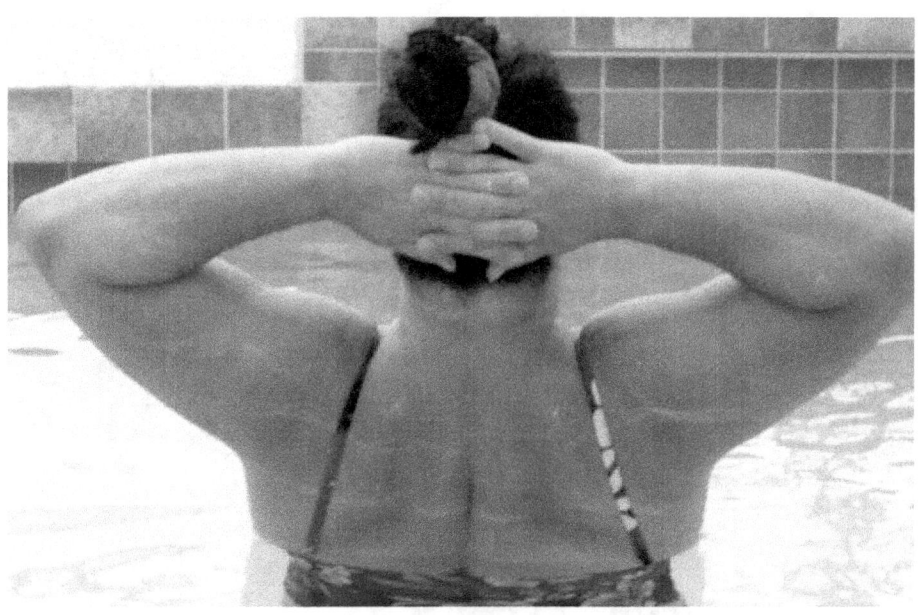

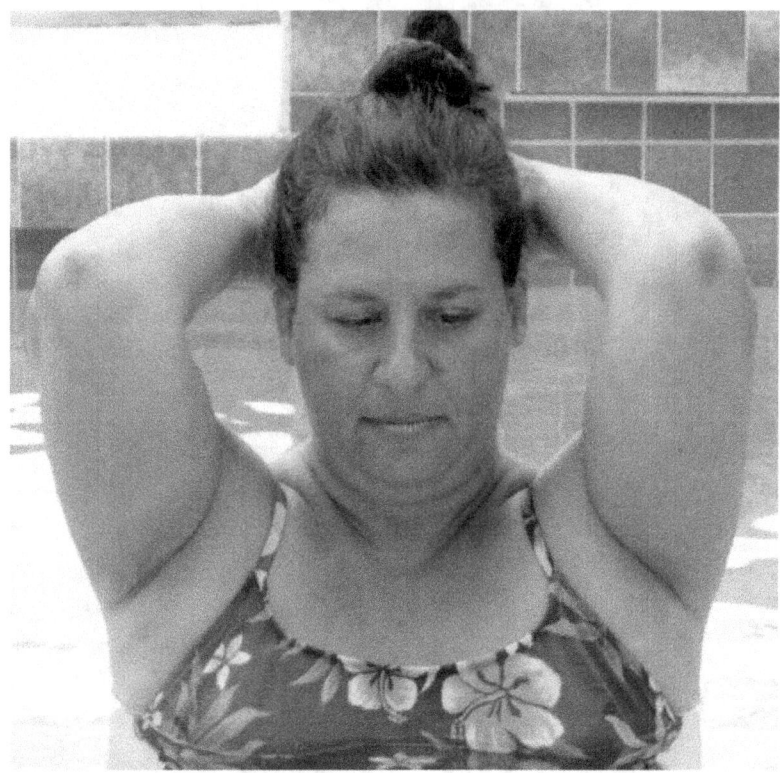

To Do:

Clasp your hands behind your head with elbows pointed outwards from the body as shown in the picture above. Now, slowly bring elbows towards the front of your body, hold, and release back to starting point. Do a total of eight repetitions.

8. Arms and Shoulders

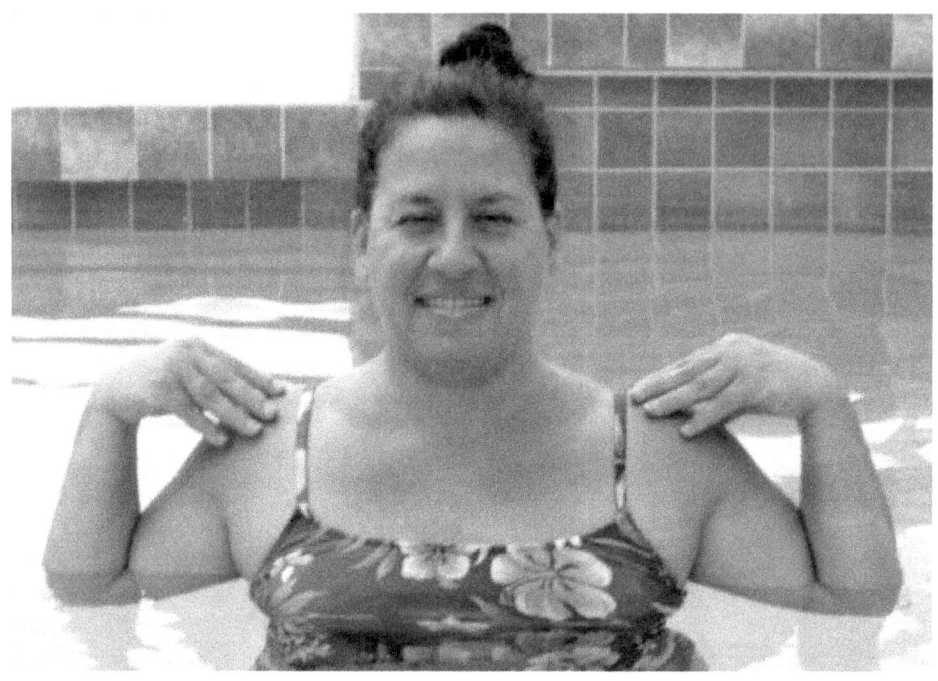

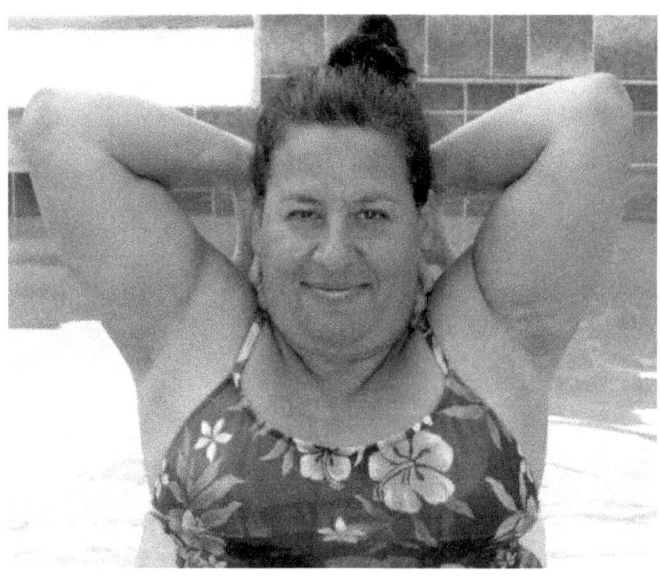

To Do:

Place your hands on your shoulder with elbows pointed downwards into the water as shown in the picture above. Now, slowly bring elbows upwards pointing to the sky, hold, and release back to starting point. Do a total of eight repetitions.

8. Arms and Shoulders

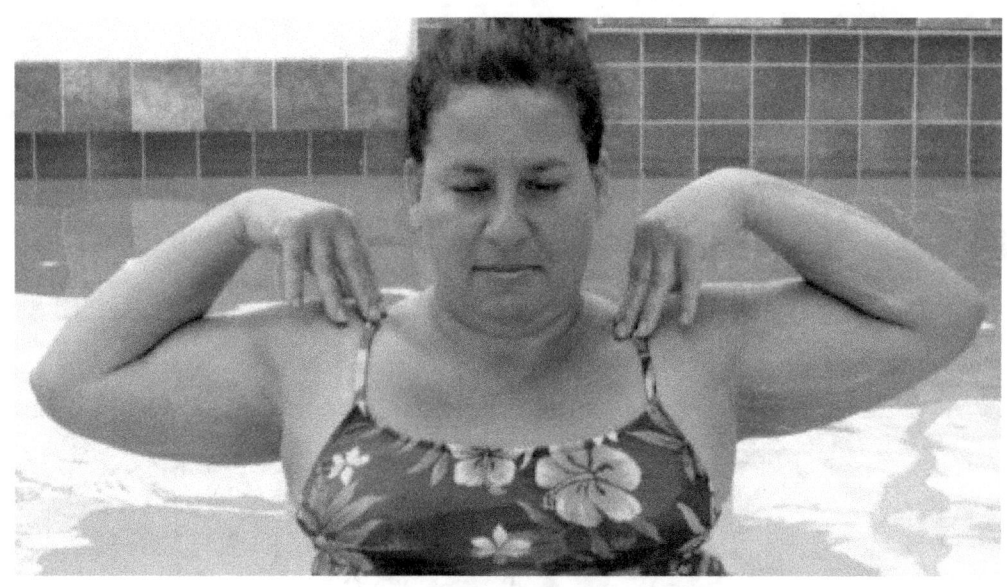

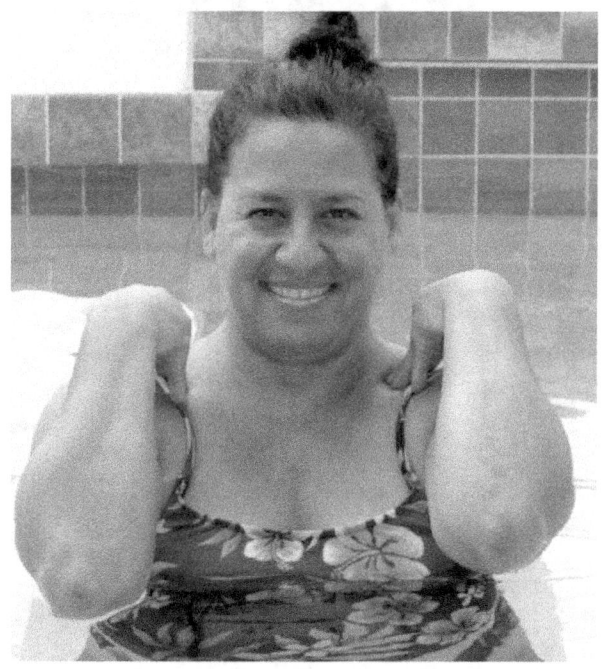

To Do:

Place your hands on your shoulder with elbows pointed outwards from your body as shown in the picture above. Now, slowly bring elbows towards the front of you body, hold, and release back to starting point. Do a total of eight repetitions.

Warm ups for the Chest and Back

1. Chest and Back

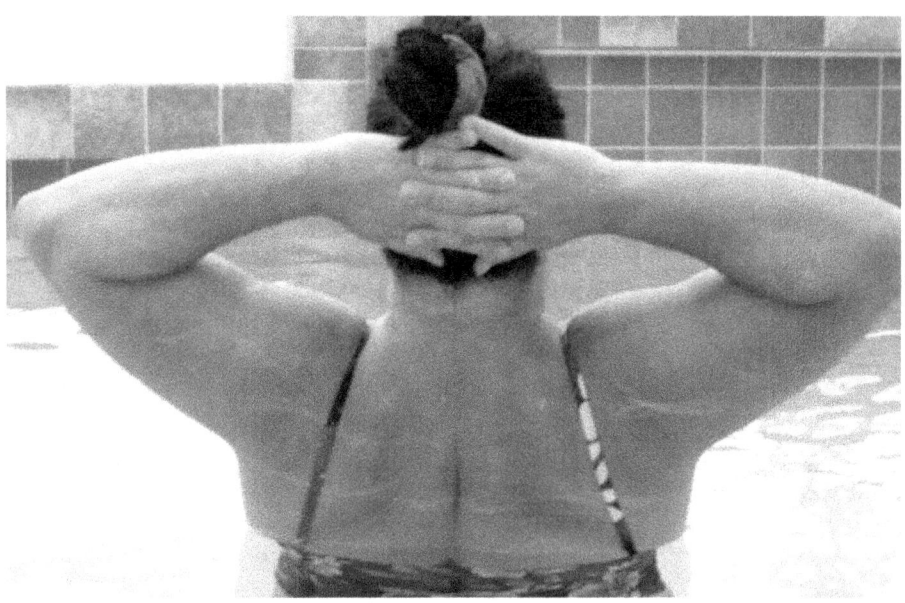

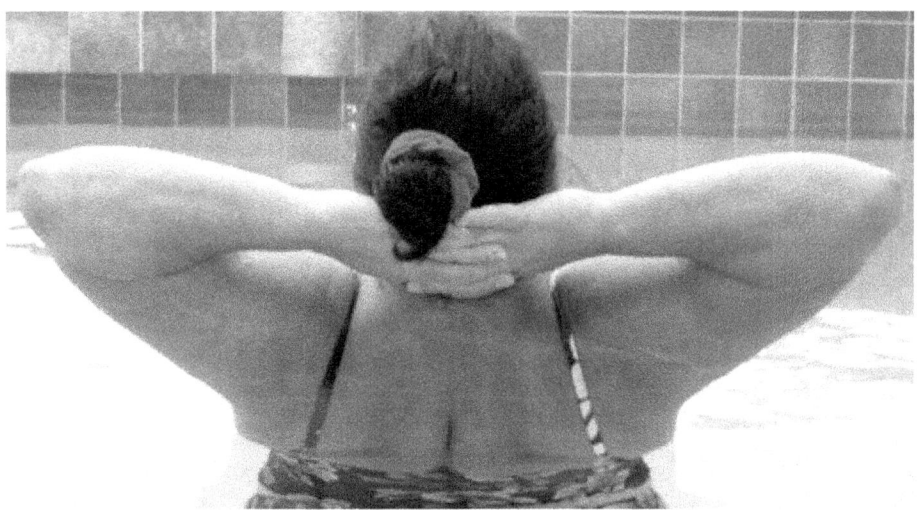

To Do:

Clasp your hands behind your head with elbows pointing away from your body as shown in the picture above. Now, slowly tilt your head backwards looking up at the sky, hold, and release back to starting point. Do a total of eight repetitions.

Hip Sway

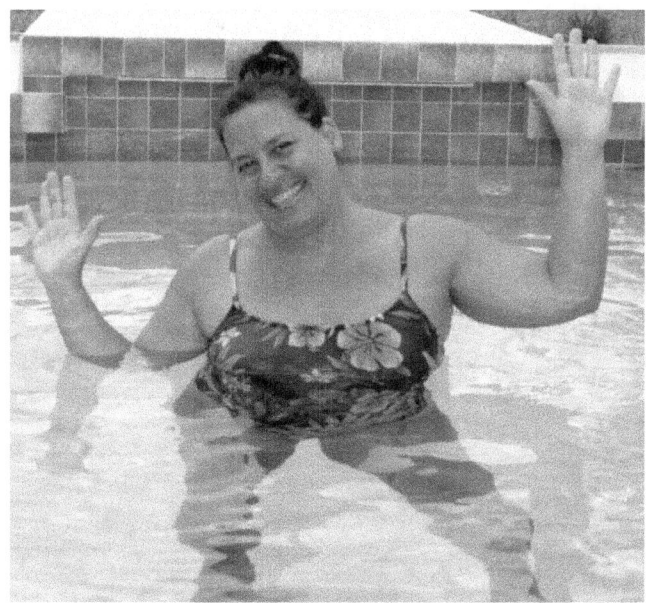 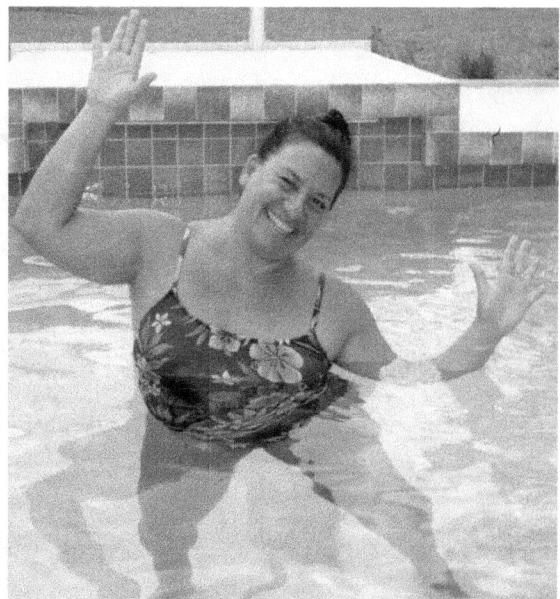

There is nothing like having a little bit of fun with your exercise routine. For the hip sway exercises listed above, you will plant both of your feet firmly on the bottom of the pool. Now, swing one hip up and to the side, then return to the center. Then, swing the other hip to the other side and return to the center.

Have fun with this exercise. Pretend you are in Hawaii and move your hips to the right and then to the left in a smooth rhythm. You can add hip bumps or change the speed of your hip sways.

To have more fun, add exciting music and use your arms to sway to the music.

Another way to loosen up the hips is to make circles in the water with your hips. Press your hips forward, to the right, towards the back, to the left, and finish back in front again. Begin with small circles and work up to large circles. Do for eight repetitions. Then reverse the direction and repeat for another eight repetitions.

You can add the belly dance hips of drawing a figure eight in front of your body. To accomplish this you will press your right hip down to the right and upward over an imaginary loop, return back to the center, press your left hip down and then upward over an imaginary loop, and return to center. Do for eight repetitions and reverse the direction and repeat for another eight repetitions.

To add variety, alternate between different moves in step with the beats of the music, or simply make it up as you go along.

1. Knee and Thigh Warm-ups

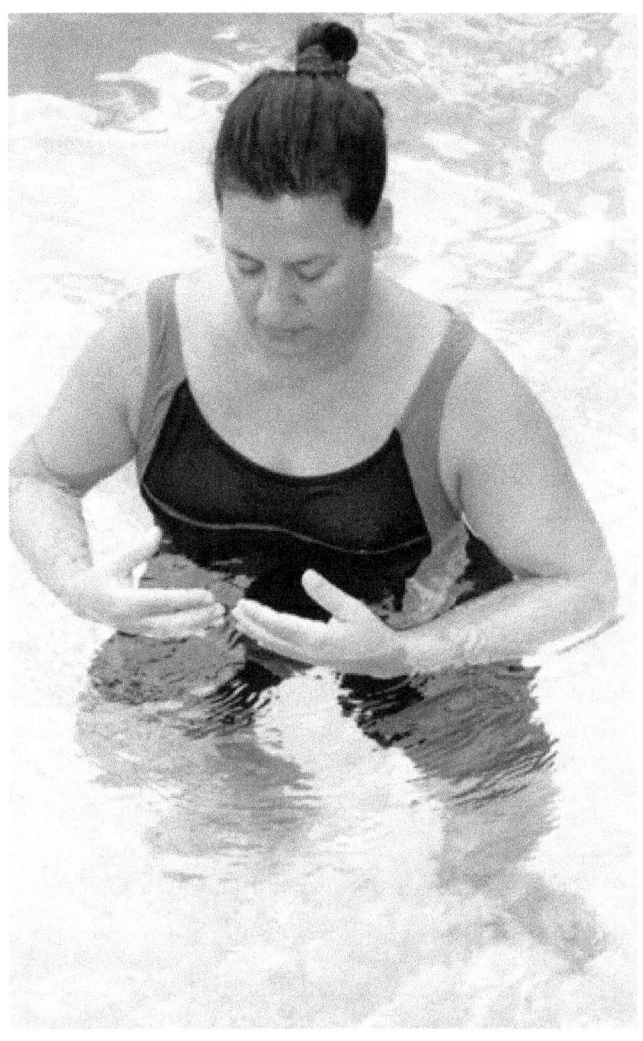

To Do:

Warm up your legs and thighs with squats. Plant both of your feet flat on the bottom of the pool and bend your knees outward as shown in the picture above. Be sure to keep your spine in a straight vertical position. This is called the Plies' squat.

Now, slowly bend your knees and allow your body to sink into the water. Remember to keep your spine perfectly straight. Do not bend forward or backward as you sink in the water.

When you have attained the position for as far down as you can sink, hold that position for a few seconds, and then release back to starting position. Repeat for eight repetitions.

Chapter Three

Basic Water Moves

1. Knee-ups

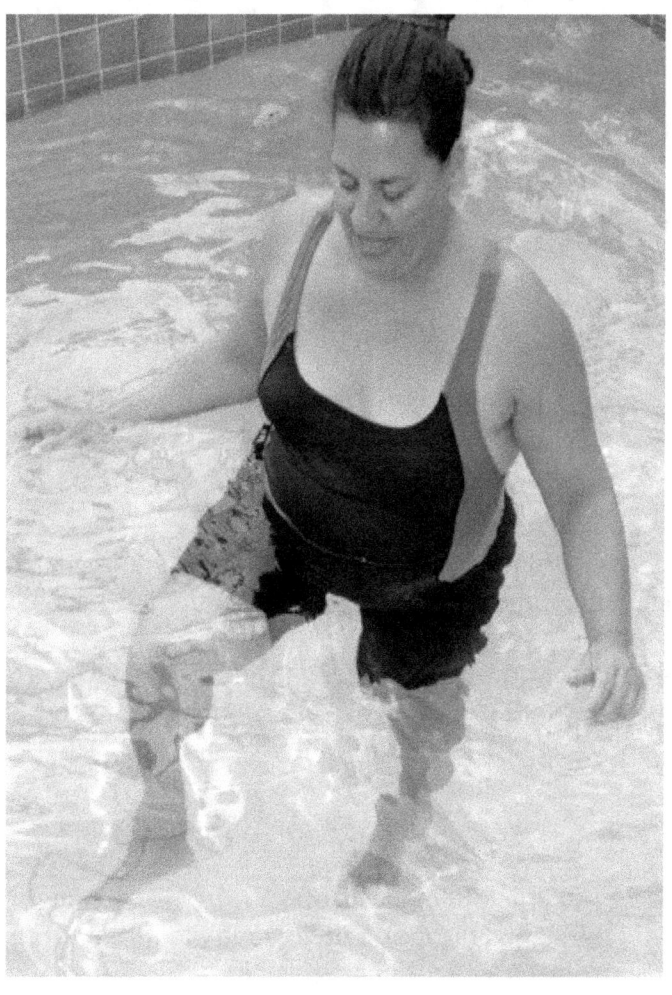

Knee-ups - Level One

Begin with both of your feet firmly planted on the bottom of the pool. Now, as you are balancing yourself, lift your right knee up as high as you can. Do not go over a 90 degree angle. Press your right foot back to the bottom of the pool and straighten out your leg. Do this for a total of 8 repetitions and repeat the whole exercise on your left leg. Work at a nice, steady, and slow speed. Take your time. Work up to 25 repetitions on each leg.

In Level One knee-ups you can also walk slowly forward and backward from one side of the pool to the other side. The faster you walk, the more intense the workout will be. In Level One you will try to keep the pace slow and steady so that you can keep your balance without too much stress on your body. I also like to make a game out of it by counting how many steps forward it takes for you to touch the side of the pool, and how many steps back it takes for you to touch the side of the pool. See if you can step wider to take fewer steps.

Knee-ups - Level Two

For Level Two, you will increase the rate of speed that you are using to lift and lower each knee. The faster you can safely lift and lower your knee, the harder the workout will be.

Walking in Level Two will be at a much faster pace now. You can call it 'Power Walking' if you like. Move your arms through the water at your side as you try to walk briskly forward and backward. Don't overdo this exercise as you will quickly discover that it will tire you out and increase your heart rate very rapidly.

Knee-ups - Level Three

There are many different facets of exercise for Level Three.

A. **Alternate Knee Lifts**

B. **Running in Place**

C. **Running with Movement**

Alternate Knee Lifts

For this exercise you will alternate between lifting the right knee and lifting the left knee. The exercise will be "Right knee up, right knee down, Left knee up, left knee down." You will repeat this for a total of 16 repetitions.

In this exercise you can also alternate the rate of speed that you are using to perform this exercise. The faster you go, the more difficult the exercise. Pace yourself and discover the right speed for you. Do not lose your body alignment to perform this exercise.

Running in Place

Should you be able to alternate the speed of your leg lifts enough, you will be able to start running in place. Do this for 30 seconds working up to a minute or more. To add variety and intensity, practice running at different rates of speed for a great workout.

Running with Movement

Now that you are up to running in place, let's add some direction. Run forward as far as you can, then run backward as far as you can. Do this for 8 repetitions.

Now, run in a clockwise circle, then shift direction and run in a counterclockwise circle. Do this for several repetitions on each side. Make the circle as large as you can so that you won't get dizzy. Should you get dizzy, stop. This is a fun time to form a Congo line if you are exercising with several other people.

2. Elbow to Knee

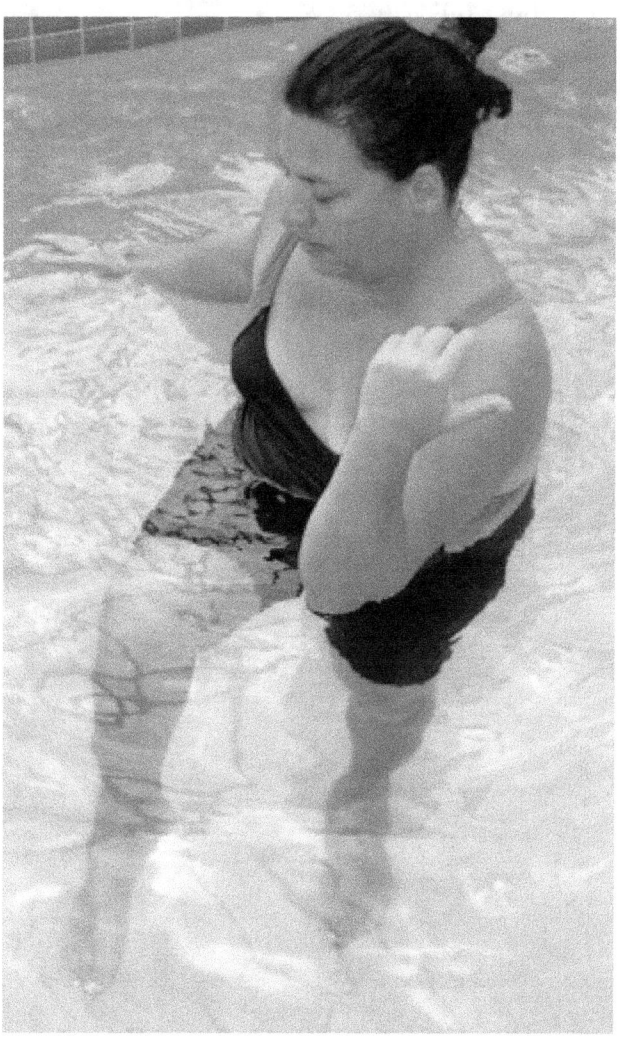

Elbow to Knee - Level One

Begin with both of your feet firmly planted on the bottom of the pool. Lift your right knee up toward the middle of the front of your body and bring your left elbow over to reach the right knee. Return the right foot back down to the bottom of the pool and straighten up your body.

Repeat bringing the right knee up and the left elbow down for a total of 8 repetitions, then repeat the entire exercise using the left knee and the right elbow.

Now, to be realistic folks, there are very few people who can really touch their knee to their elbow. So, I don't want you to think that this is what you have to do in order to do this exercise correctly. As long as your knee is coming across to the front of your body and you are bringing your left elbow down towards that knee, you are doing the exercise correctly.

Please, do don't strain yourself to get these body parts to touch and do don't twist so much as to hurt your back. Your muscles will loosen up over time and you will notice in a matter weeks that you are don't straining anymore. The exercise will feel easier the more you practice it, I promise you.

Be sure to make your movements slow and deliberate. Do not throw your body out of alignment or contort your body needlessly. Inhale as you straighten and exhale as you bring the elbow to the knee. Work up to 25 repetitions on each knee.

Elbow to Knee - Level Two

In Level Two you will do the same exercise but you will alternate the elbow to the knees. The exercise will go like this: "Left elbow to Right knee, straighten up, Right elbow to left knee, and straighten up. You will do this for a total of 16 repetitions. Work up to 25 repetitions.

Elbow to Knee - Level Three

You will now do the alternate elbow to knee lifts as described in Level Two but at a faster rate of speed. You will feel like you are running and feet may not come fully down on the bottom of the pool. To add variety and intensity, alternate between slow and fast rates of speed, this will help to build up your heart rate. If you like, you can move forward and backward while doing this exercise.

3. Touch Foot in Front

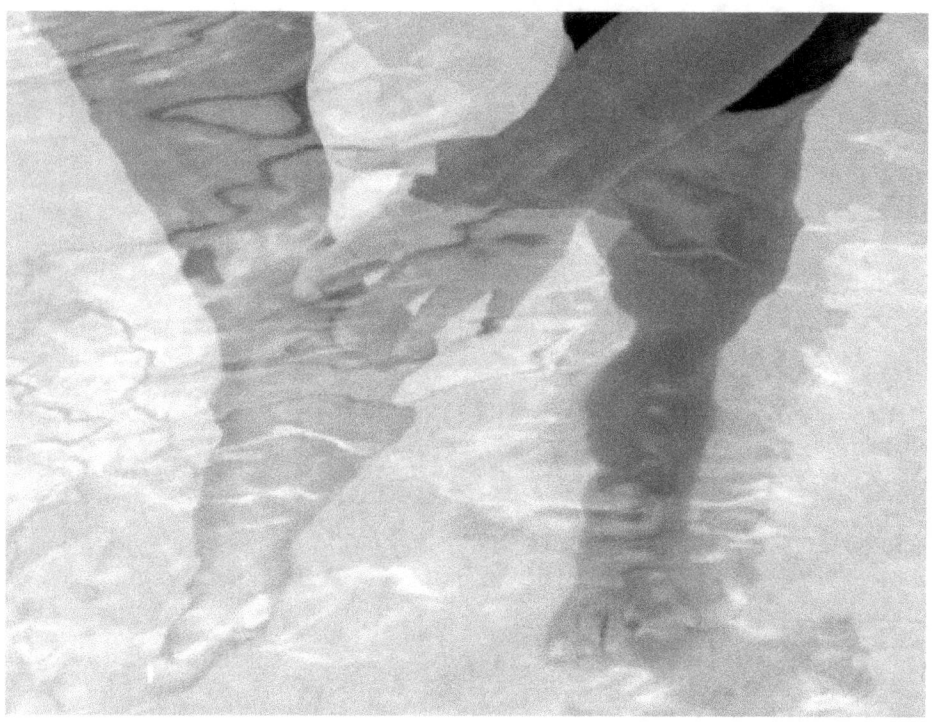

Touch Foot in Front - Level One

For this exercise you will bring your right foot up in front of your body and you will reach down into the water with your left hand to touch the right foot. Straighten up and repeat again bringing your right foot up to the front of your body and touching it with your left hand. Repeat this exercise for at least 8 repetitions, building to 25.

When finished, repeat this exercising bringing your left up in front of your body and reaching down with your right hand to touch your foot. Straighten up and repeat the exercise again for a total of 8 repetitions, building to 25. Keep a nice, slow and steady pace. If you can't touch your foot, that is alright. Just do the best that you can.

Touch Foot in Front - Level Two

To add intensity to movement described in level two we will alternated the feet. The directions will be as follows: "Right foot up, left hand down, Left foot up, right hand down."

You can also increase the intensity of this movement by adding speed creating a hopping effect from foot to foot. The faster you go, the higher the intensity. Repeat for 16 to 25 repetitions.

4. Touch Foot in Back

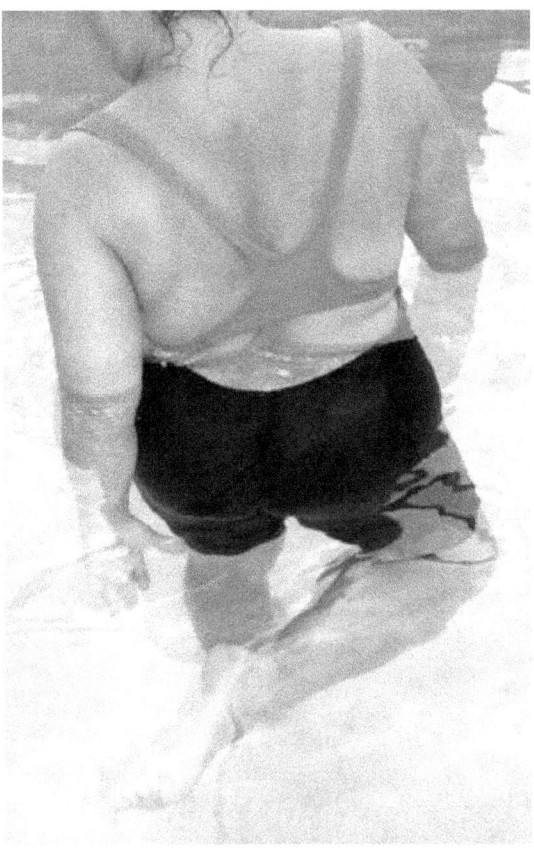

Touch Foot in Back - Level One

Just like the exercise listed before it, back you will perform this exercise to the back of your body. Bring your right foot up behind your body and reach down into the water with your left hand and try to touch your foot, straighten up your body, and repeat the exercise again on the same foot for 8 repetitions. Build up to 25 repetitions. When finished, repeat the entire exercise using your left foot and your right hand. Do not strain or twist your back in order to do these exercises. Do what is comfortable for you.

Please note that you do not have to actually touch your foot in order to derive some benefits from this exercise. Just do the best that you can do.

Touch Foot in Back - Level Two

To build intensity in this movement you can begin by alternating the left foot and right hand and right foot and left hand. The directions will be: "Left foot up, right hand down, Right foot up, left hand down." Repeat for 16 to 25 repetitions.

To increase the intensity of this exercise even more, add speed to the movements. You will feel like you are hopping from one foot to the other. You can also add varying speeds to this exercise to make it feel more intense.

5. Front Leg Lifts

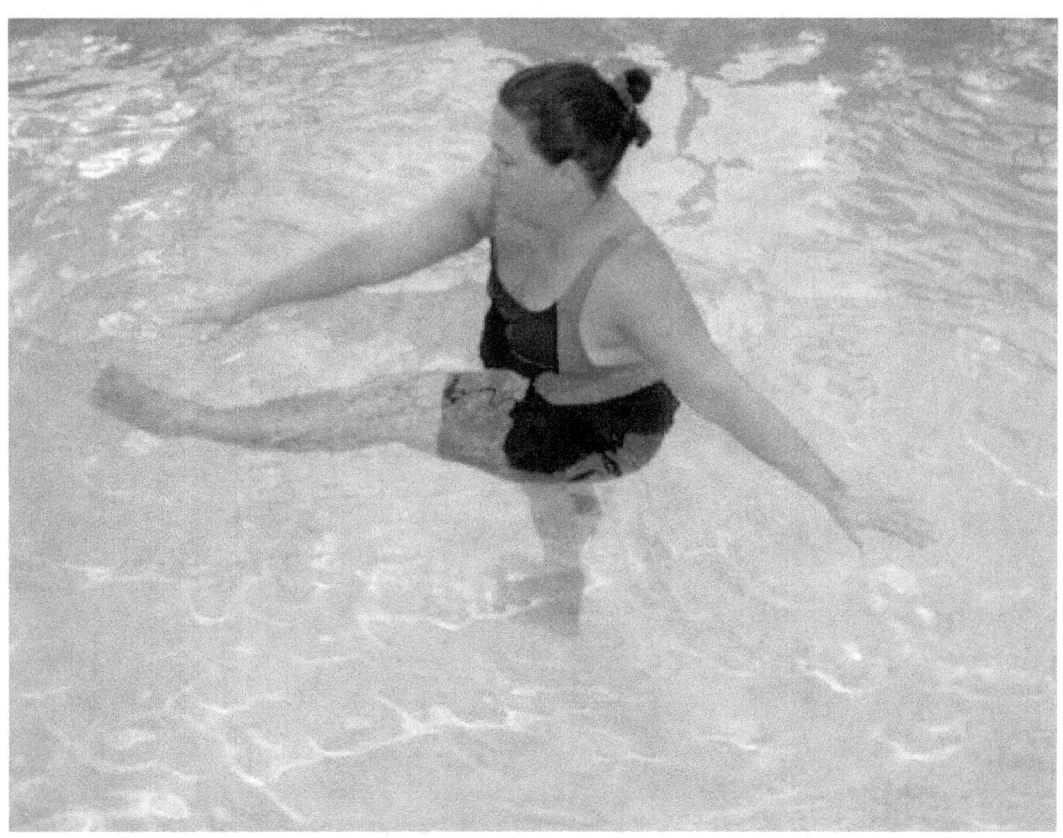

Front Leg Lifts – Level One

Begin with both feet planted firmly on the bottom of the pool and with your knees soft. Now, inhale and bring your left leg straight up in front of you as high as you comfortably can, hold for a few seconds, and then as exhale, bring your leg back down to the starting position. Repeat for a total of eight repetitions.

When finished, repeat the entire exercise with your right leg for a total of eight repetitions.

Front Leg Lifts - Level Two

Begin in the starting position listed above. This time you will alternate lifting your left leg and returning it to the starting position and then lifting your right leg and returning it to the starting position. Continue alternative the front leg lifts for a total of 16 repetitions.

Front Leg Lifts – Level Three

Repeat this exercise as listed in Level Two only add speed, hopping from right to left leg. You can also move forward and backward while alternating front leg lifts.

6. Side Leg Lifts

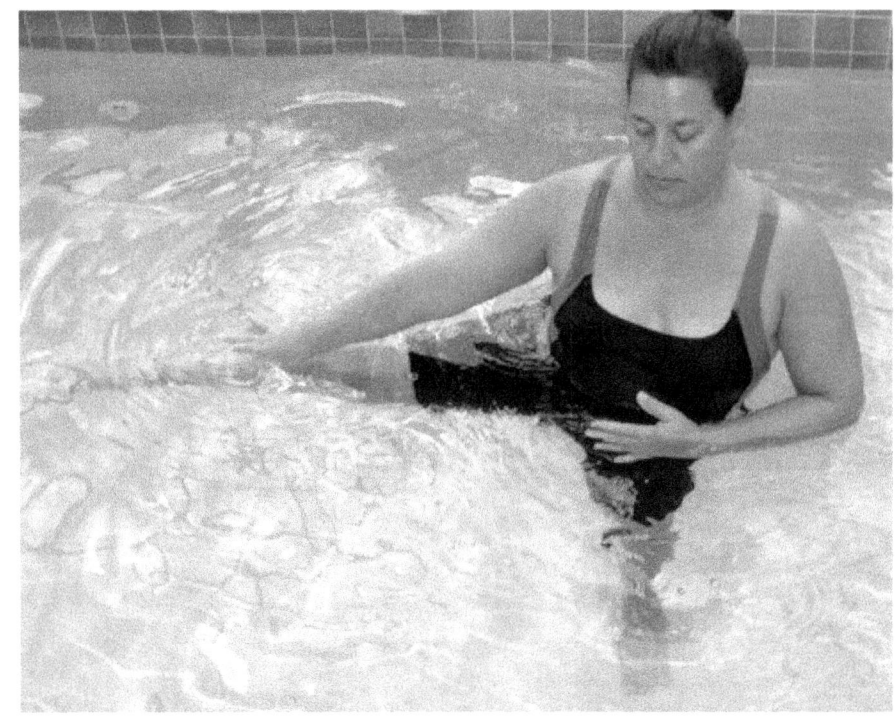

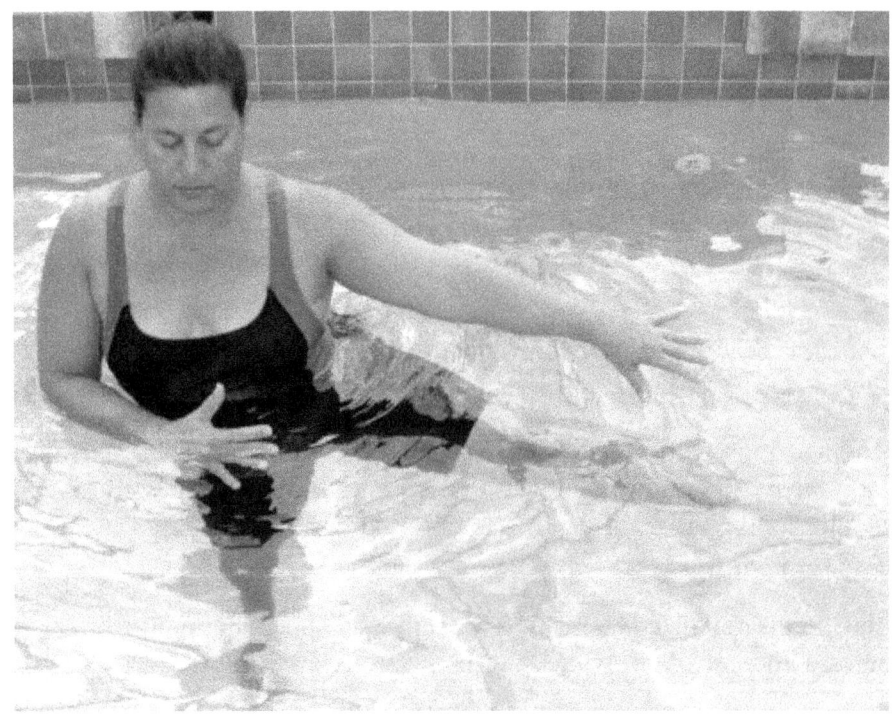

Side Leg Lifts – Level One

Plant both of your feet firmly on the bottom of the pool and keep your knees soft. Now, inhale and lift your right straight up at your side as high as you comfortably can, hold for a few seconds, and then exhale and release the leg back to the starting position. Repeat for a total of eight repetitions.

When finished, repeat the entire exercise on your left leg for a total of eight repetitions.

Side Leg Lifts - Level Two

Plant both of your feet firmly on the bottom of the pool and keep your knees soft. Now, lift your right leg up as far as you can to your right side and return to the starting position. Then, lift your left leg up as far as you can to your left side and return to the starting position. Repeat alternating between the right leg and the left leg for a total of 16 repetitions.

Side Leg Lifts – Level Three

In this exercise you will complete the side kicks as described in level two only you add speed to the exercise shifting rapidly between the right and left leg lifts. You can also move forward and backward as you do this exercise.

As an added treat, do this exercise while moving sideways from one end of the pool to the other. You can vary your speed and even add a double hop on one foot to add variety to your workout.

Play some upbeat music while you are exercising and 'dance' to the music while you are doing your water workout. Match your speed and movements to the songs you have chosen to alleviate any boredom you may suffer from exercise.

With music, you see the time fly by very quickly. Be sure to pick music that makes you want to move and if you can sing along with the words, all the better.

7. Inner/Outer Thigh Work

NOTE: Do not cross the midline of the body if you have had a hip replacement.

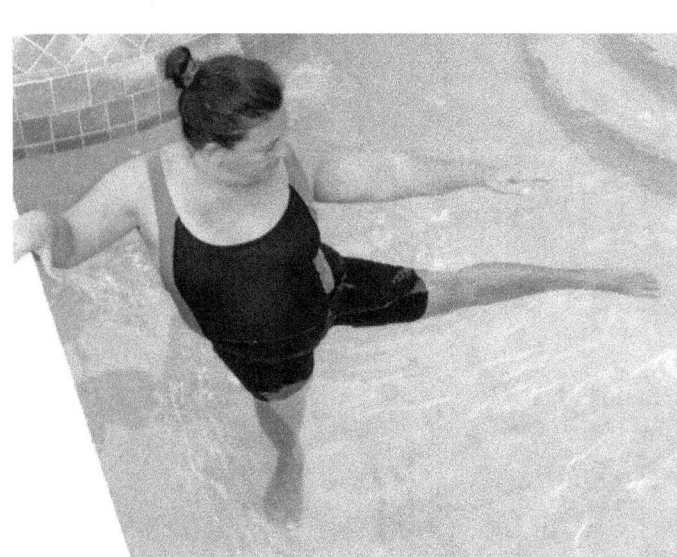 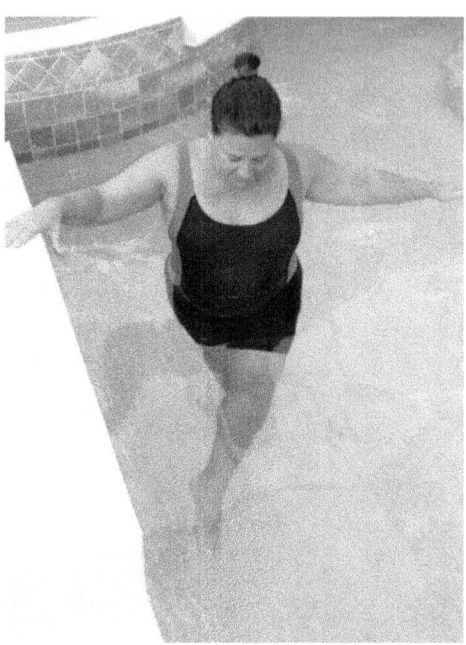

Begin by planting both feet firmly on the bottom of the pool and softening your knees. You are encouraged to hold on to the side of the pool while performing this exercise.

Inhale and lift your left leg as high as you comfortably can straight out from the side of your body, hold for a few seconds, and as you exhale bring the leg back towards your body and sweep it front of your right leg. Inhale and bring the leg back up to the side of your body as high as you comfortably can and as you exhale, sweep that leg in front of your standing leg. Repeat for a total of eight repetitions.

When finished, turn around in the pool and face the opposite direction. This time you will inhale and bring the right leg up as high as you comfortably can at the side of your body and as you exhale you will sweep that leg in front of your left, standing leg. Repeat for a total of eight repetitions.

8. Lunges

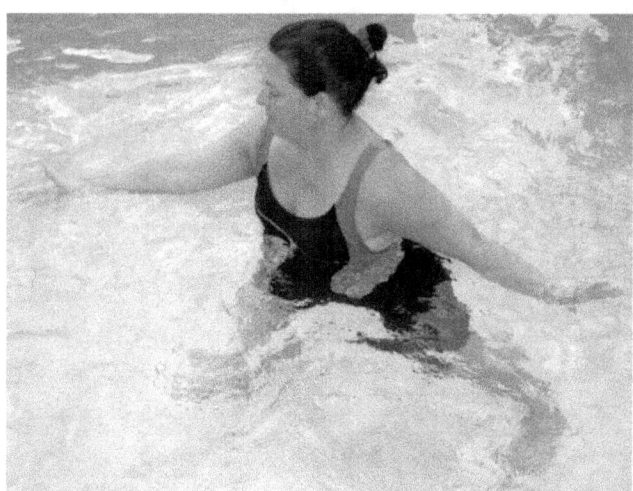 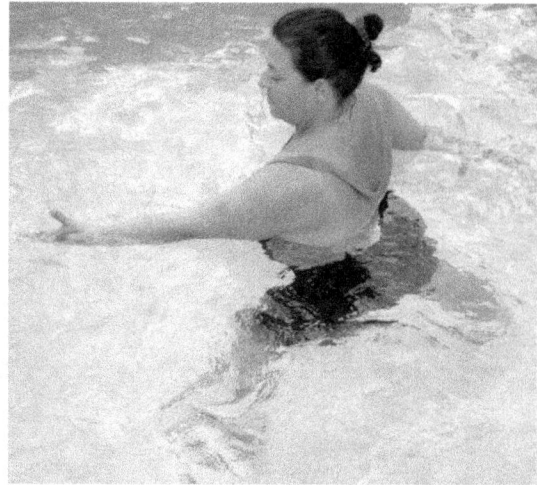

Lunges – Level One

Begin with both feet planted firmly on the bottom of the pool with your knees soft. Now, as you jump up from the bottom of the pool, bring your right leg forward and your left leg back.

As you land on the bottom of the pool, your right foot should be planted firmly in front of you and your left foot should be directly behind you (landing on the ball of your foot-not flat).

Now, jump up from the bottom of the pool again and this time bring your left foot in front of you and bring your right foot behind you. Repeat this jumping up from the bottom of the pool and switching one leg in front of your body and the other leg behind your body. Continue for a total of 16 repetitions, eight on each leg.

Lunges - Level Two

For level two, you will perform the exercise as listed in level one only you will add speed to the movement. The faster you switch your legs, the harder and more intense the exercise will become.

You can also add variety to the movement by staying in the lunge position for a double count and then switching legs rapidly for a six count. Continue for a total of 16 repetitions. Have fun with this movement and make it as challenging as you would like.

9. Jumping Jacks

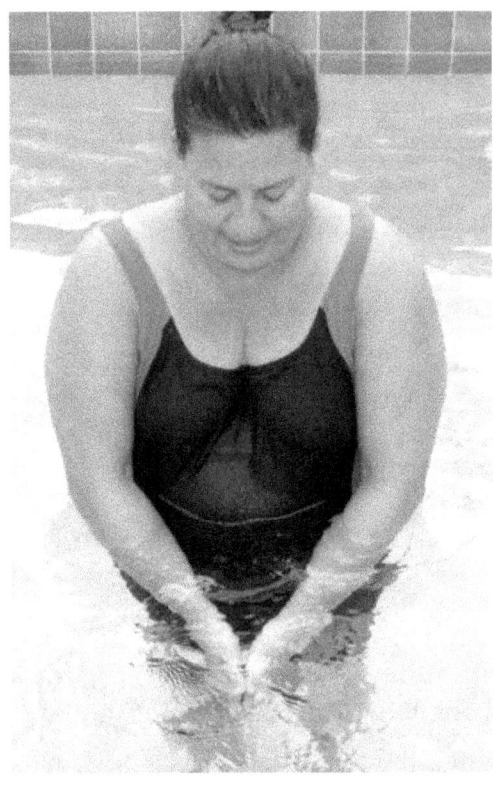

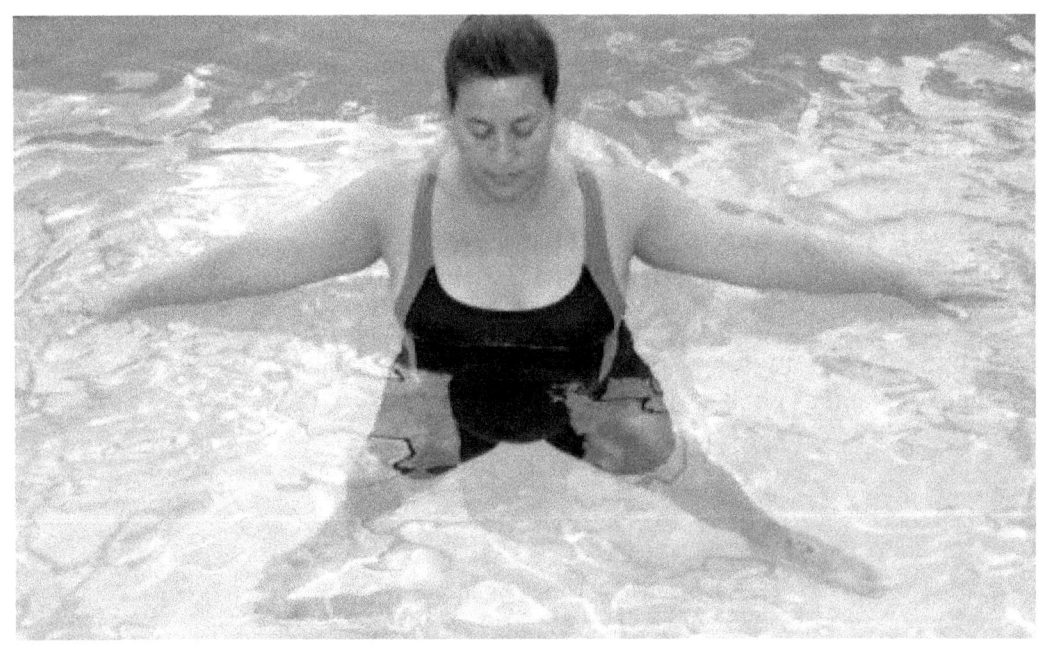

Jumping Jacks – Level One

Begin with both of your feet planted firmly on the bottom of the pool with your knees soft. Bring both of your hands together in front of you and in the water. You will keep your hands IN the water through out this entire exercise.

Inhale and jump up from the bottom of the pool and spread your legs out to both sides of your body. As you separate your legs, separate your arms out to your sides as well.

Exhale and jump up from the bottom of the pool and bring both of your legs and arms back together again as in the starting position above. Continue jumping out and in for a total of eight repetitions.

Jumping Jacks - Level Two

Repeat the same exercise as described above only add speed to the jumping jacks. The faster you jump out and back in, the more intense the workout will be.

You may also add movement to this exercise. You can move forward and backward if you like. I like to do this exercise facing all four corners of the pool.

I have found that making a game out of it keeps me interested and working. I usually begin by facing one end of the pool and I do five jumping jacks and at the end of the fifth jumping jack I jump up and make a 90 degree turn to the right. I then do another 5 jumping jacks and after the fifth jumping jack I jump up and make a 90 degree turn. I continue until I have gone all around the pool. When I find myself back where I started, I do five jumping jacks and then after the fifth one I reverse by direction by jumping up and making a 90 degree turn to the left and repeat the exercise going the other way. Doing the exercise this way I can take in my surroundings which is then always changing keeping me interested in the workout that I am doing. I like to break up the tedious of exercising in this way.

10. Hamstring Curls

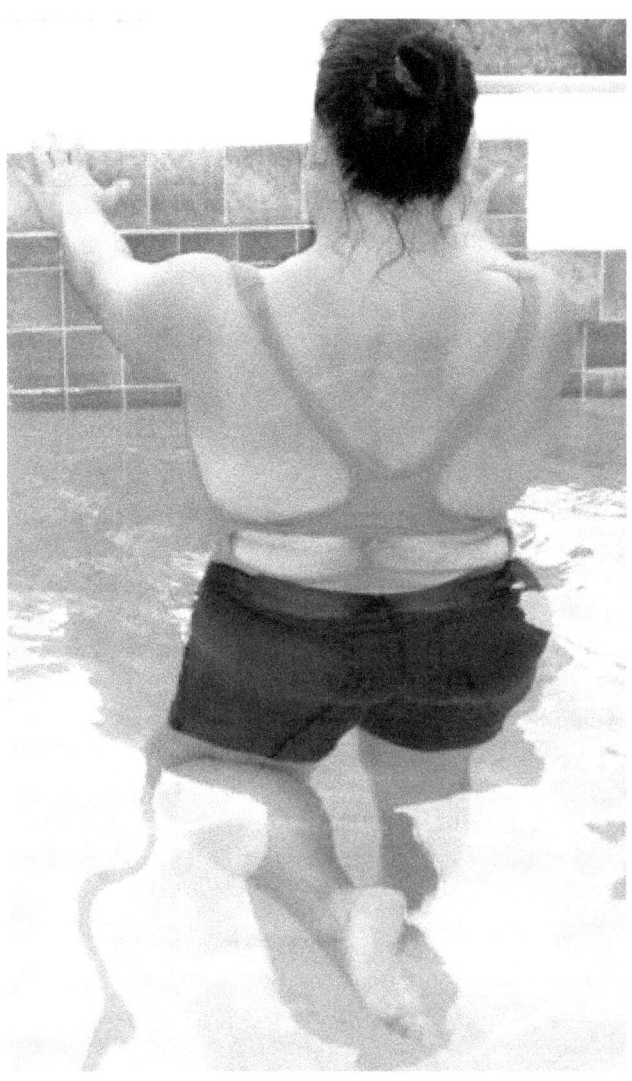

Level One

Begin with both of your feet planted firmly on the bottom of the pool with your knees soft. You may hold on to the side of the pool for support.

Inhale and bring the heel of your left up towards your left buttocks, hold for a few seconds, and as you exhale bring the left foot back down to the bottom of the pool Repeat for a total of 8 repetitions.

Repeat this exercise by bringing the heel of your right foot to your right buttocks. Repeat for a total of eight repetitions.

Level Two

Repeat the exercise above but this time alternate between the left foot and the right foot. Add speed and movement to increase the intensity of this exercise.

Chapter Four

Stretches

1. Shoulder Stretch

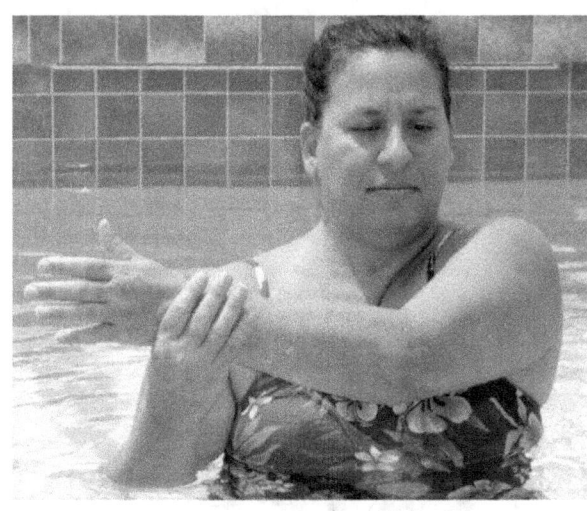 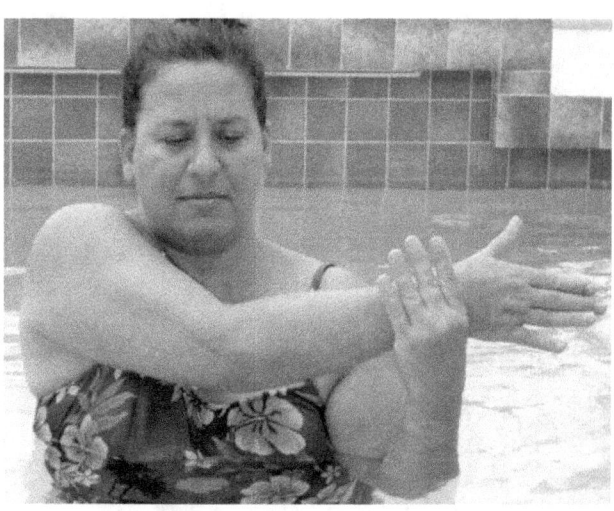

1   2

Begin the cool down by bring your straight left arm across the front of your body and gently grasp your left wrist with your right hand (as shown in picture #1). Gently press the left arm toward your right arm.

Be sure to keep your hips and body straight and looking forward. Do not force the stretch and be sure to inhale and exhale freely and easily. Release the arm.

Now, take your straight right arm and bring it across the front of your body and gently grasp your right wrist with your left hand and press the arms towards your left arm (as shown in picture #2).

Release the arm. Repeat on both sides for an additional two more times.

2. Shoulder Hug

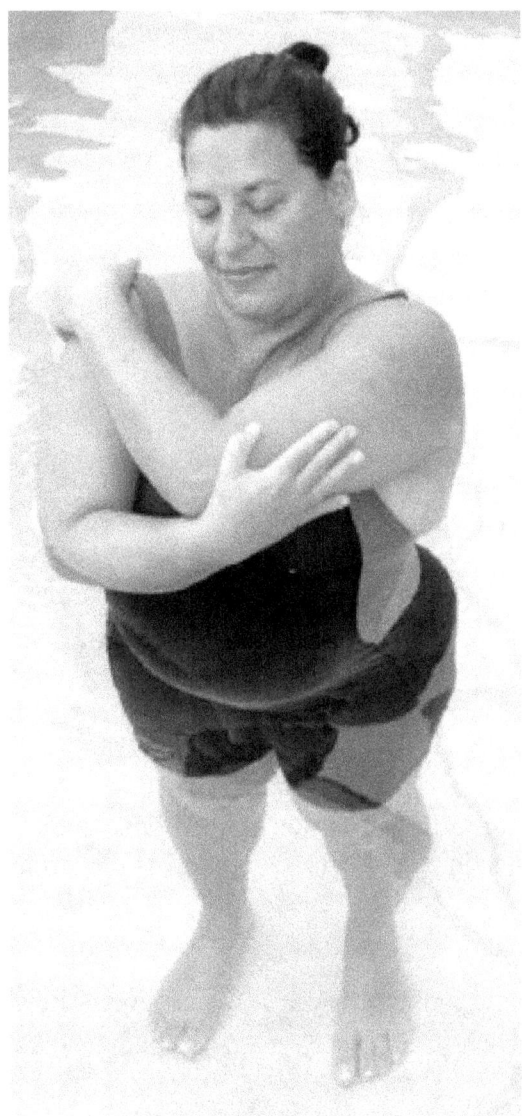 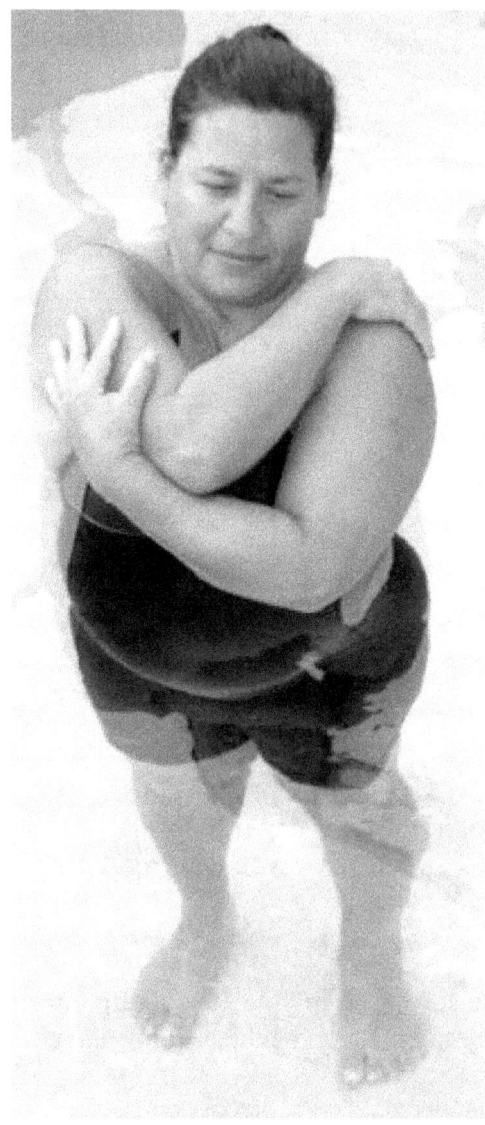

A great shoulder stretch in the 'hug'. Just wrap your arms around each other and give yourself a big hug. Inhale and exhale freely and easily.

Release your hug and switch your arms around and give yourself another big hug. Inhale and exhale freely and easily.

Repeat the hug for an additional two more times on each side.

3. Tricep Stretch

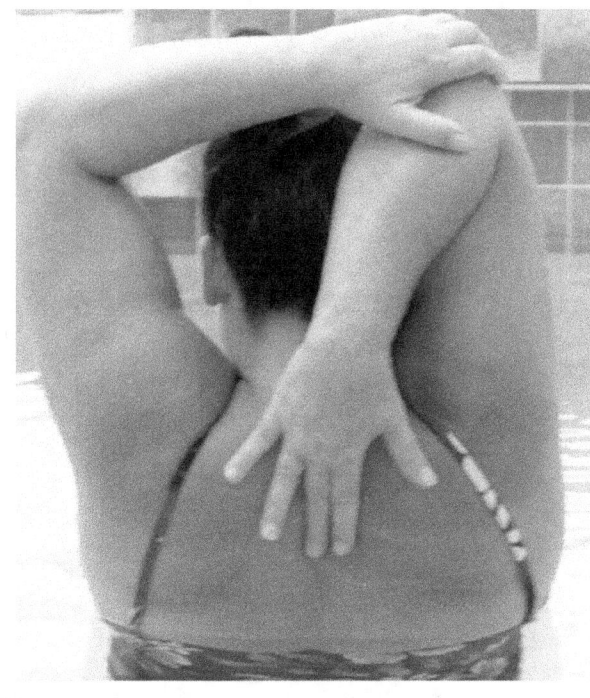

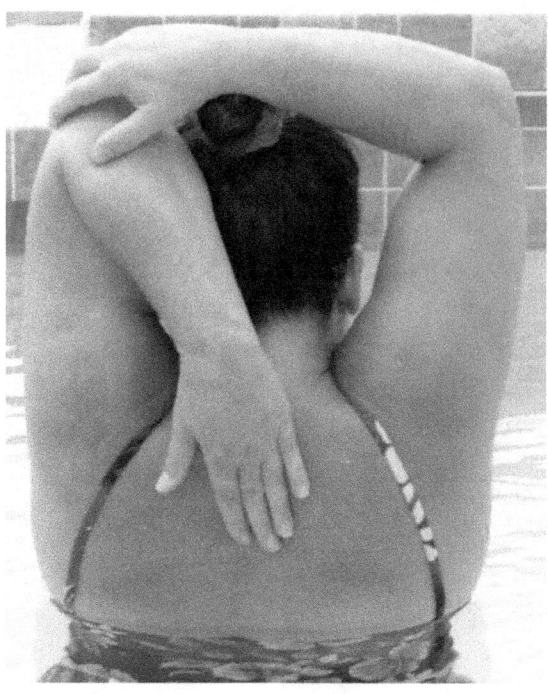

1

2

Bring your right arm straight out in front of your body and reach upward. Bend the elbow and bring the right hand down to lay flat on your back with the palm of your right hand on your back.

Bring your left hand over and place it on your right elbow. Gently add pressure to your right elbow to push it backward giving you a stretch in your triceps muscle. Breathe normally.

Release your arm and bring your left arm straight out in front of your body and reach upward. Bend the elbow and bring the left hand down to lay palms flat on your back.

Bring your right hand over and place it on your left elbow. Gently add pressure to your left elbow and push it backward giving you a stretch in your triceps muscle. Breathe normally. Continue stretching the tricep for an additional two more times.

4. Lat Stretch

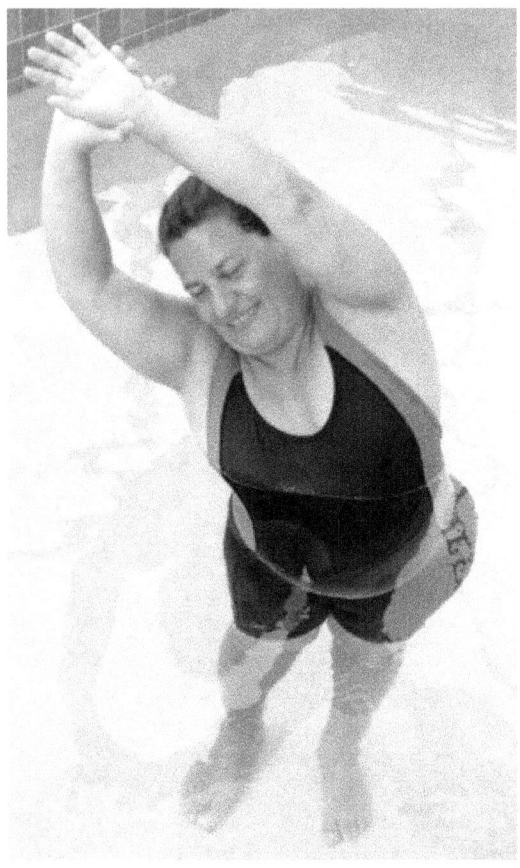

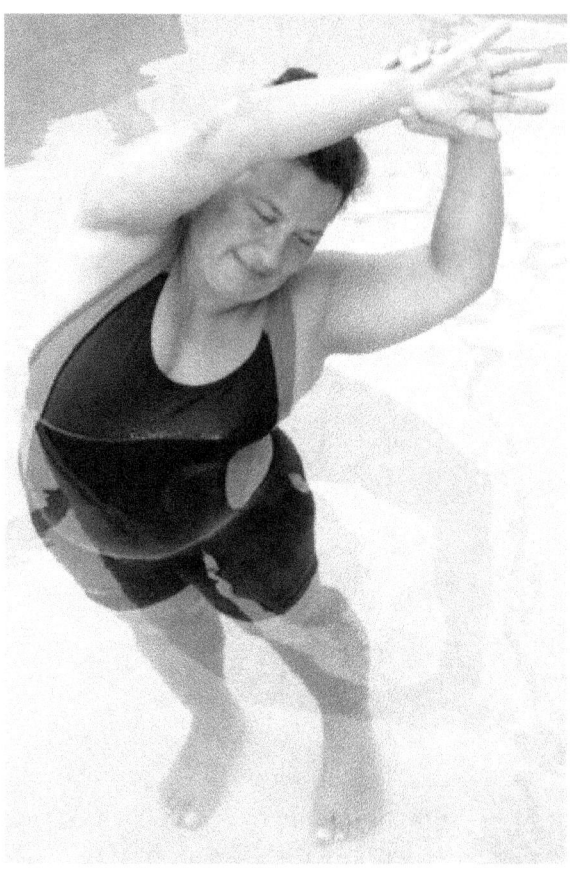

1   2

     Begin this exercise by standing with feet flat on the bottom of the pool and shoulder width apart. Reach your left arm straight upward from your body. Inhale and clasp your left wrist with your right hand. As you exhale, gently pull the left hand, and arm, down towards the right. Inhale and return to starting position and exhale and release.

     Inhale again. This time extend your right arm straight upward from your body. Inhale and clasp your right wrist with your left hand. As you exhale, gently pull the right hand, and arm, down towards the left. Inhale and return to starting position and exhale and release.

Repeat this exercise for a total of at least 8 stretches on each side of the body.

5. Hip Stretch

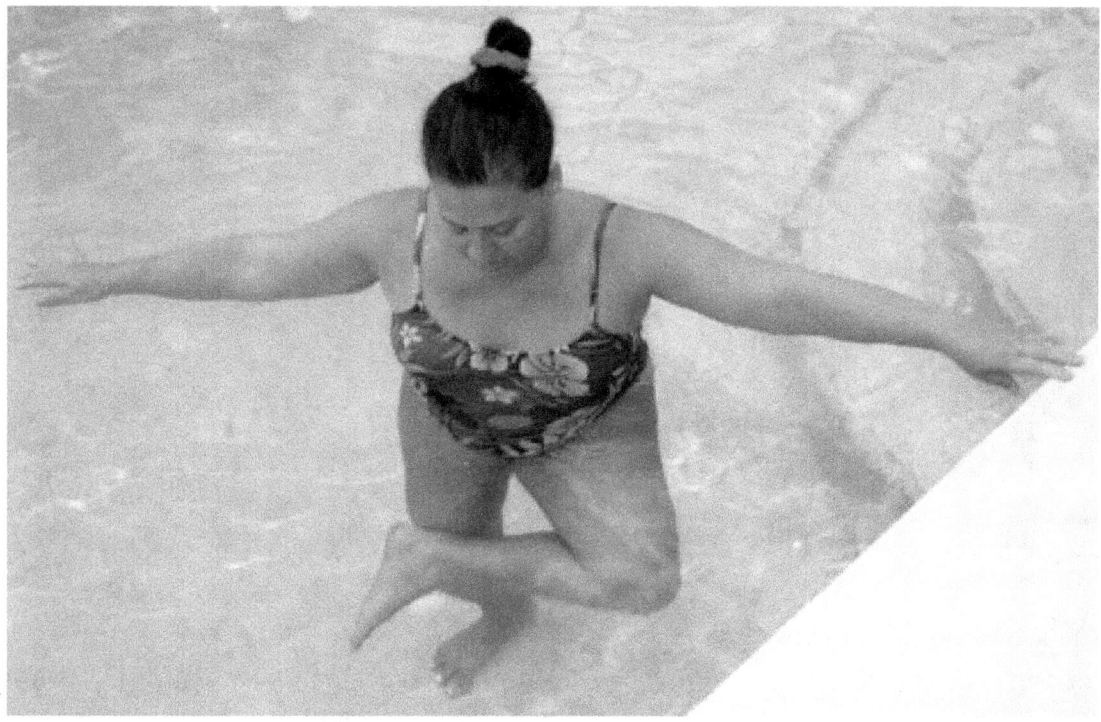

Begin this exercise by standing with both of your feet planted firmly on the bottom of the pool shoulder width apart. Bend your left knee and bring your left up the front of your body and place it just above your knee.

Now, as you exhale, slowly bend your right knee and allow yourself to sink into the water as far as you can comfortably go. Hold, and then release into starting position. Repeat this exercise on the other side using your right foot on your left thigh.

To add more depth to this hip stretch exercise you can do the following: As you sink into the water as far down as you can go, hold that position and lift up off the heel of your foot.

To add balance to this exercise, try to do this exercise without holding on to the side of the pool. This may be very difficult to do depending upon the water flow in your pool.

7. Back Stretch

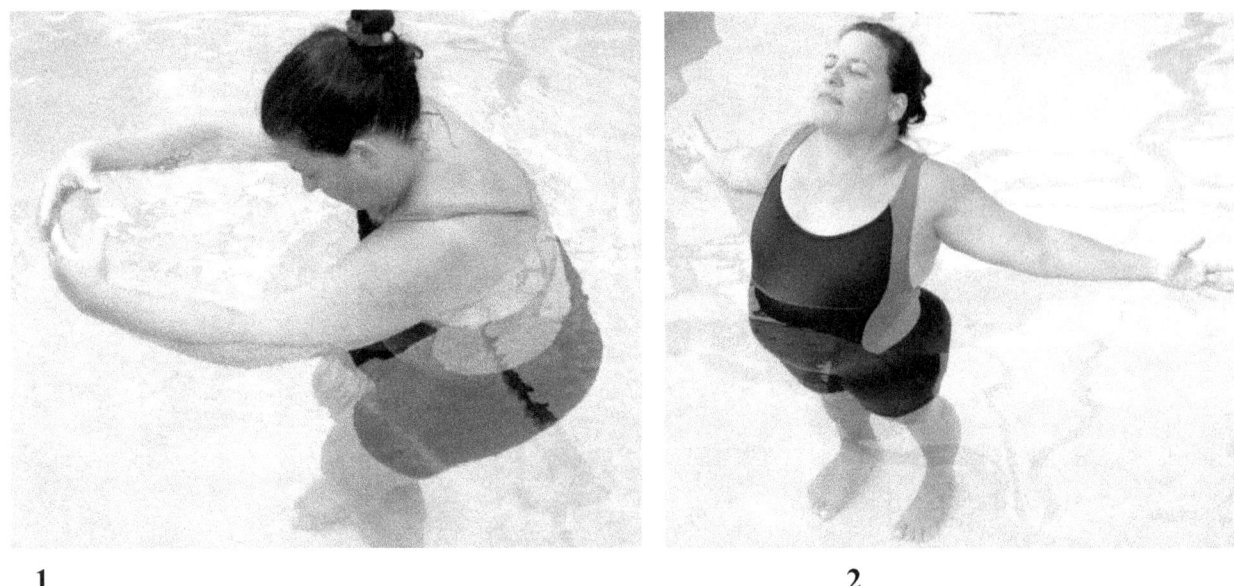

1   2

Begin this exercise by standing with your feet firmly planted on the bottom of the pool shoulder width apart. Inhale, and as you exhale, bend your knees and slowly arch your back forward as shown in the Diagram #1.

As you inhale, stand up straight and arch your back slightly backwards. Let your arms open wide from your sides opening up your chest as much as you comfortably can as shown in Diagram #2.

When you exhale, roll yourself into the position as shown in Diagram #1.

Repeat this exercise for at least three good deep breaths.

8. Side Stretch

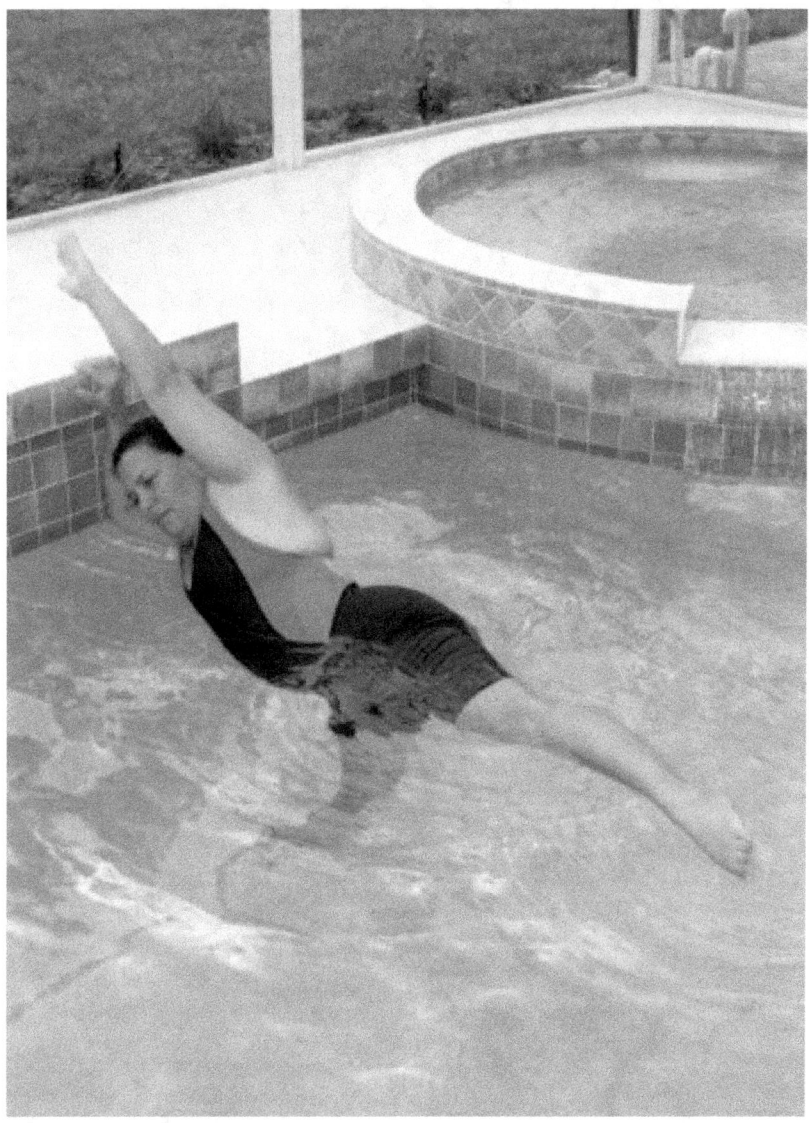

Begin by standing with your feet firmly planted on the bottom of the pool about shoulder width apart. Stand with the fingers of your right hand touching the side of the pool.

Inhale and bend your right elbow, lifting your right arm straight upwards. As you exhale, bring the right arm over your head and lift your left leg straight out from the side of your body. Feel a good full body stretch, hold, and release back into starting position.

Repeat the exercise on this side of the body for a total of eight repetitions before turning around and performing this exercise on the other side of your body.

9. Body Stretch

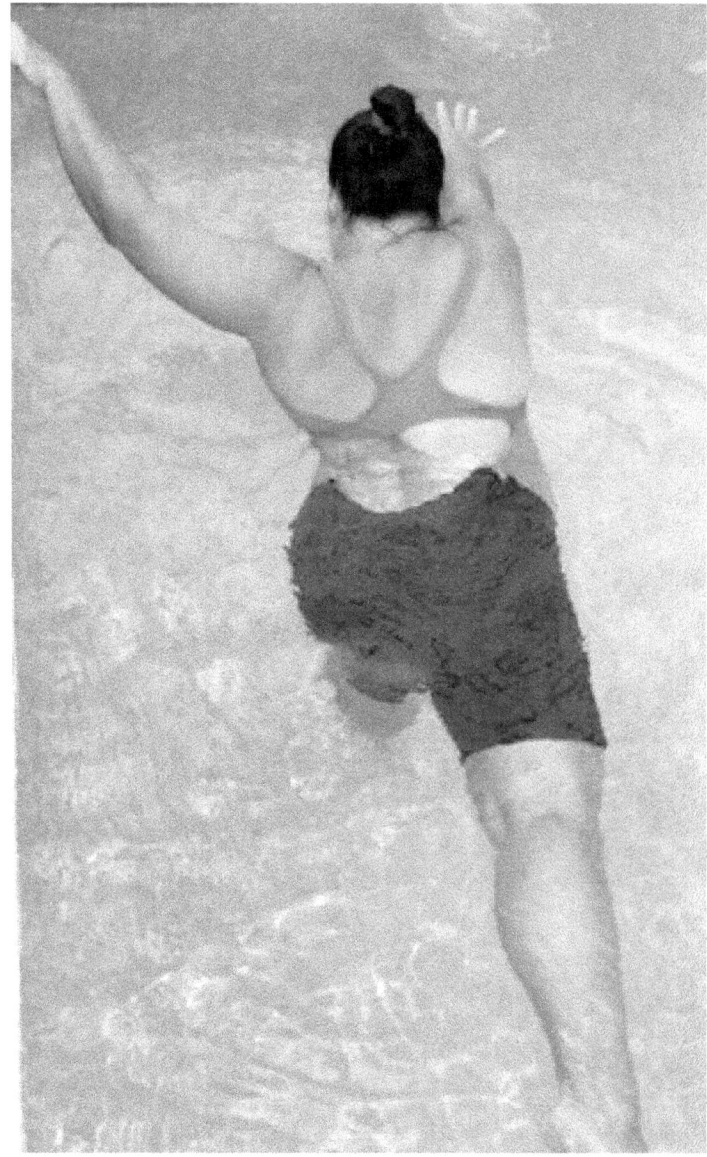

Start with your feet planted firmly on the bottom of the pool shoulder width apart. Inhale and extend your right arm straight upwards. As you exhale, bend your torso and the right arm to the front as close to the top of the water line as you can get. Extend your right leg straight back behind you pointing your toes.

Inhale and return to the starting position. Repeat this exercise for a total of eight repetitions on the right side of your body before turning around and repeating this exercise on the other side of your body. To add intensity to this exercise, try to perform this exercise without holding on to the side of the pool.

Chapter Five

Balance and Cool Down

Balance-Yoga Style

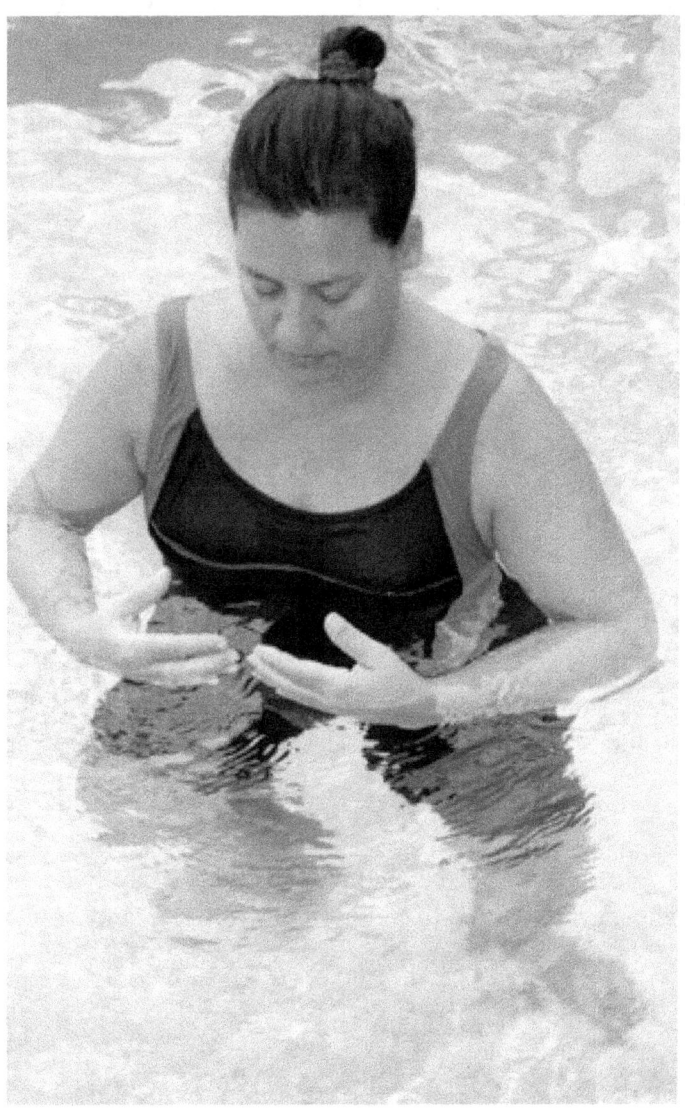

This is a great exercise movement to help strengthen the core of your body while improving your balance and focus. Stand with feet planted firmly on the bottom of the pool at shoulder width apart. Bend both of your knees slightly outward at the sides. Bring both of your hands out in front of your body at just below heart level (should be just below the top of the water line). The palms of both hands are facing in towards the front of your torso.

Find a focal point and allow your mind to sit in that focal point. Inhale and exhale smoothly, slowly and deeply. Try to clear your mind of all outside annoyances and distractions. Enjoy the moment.

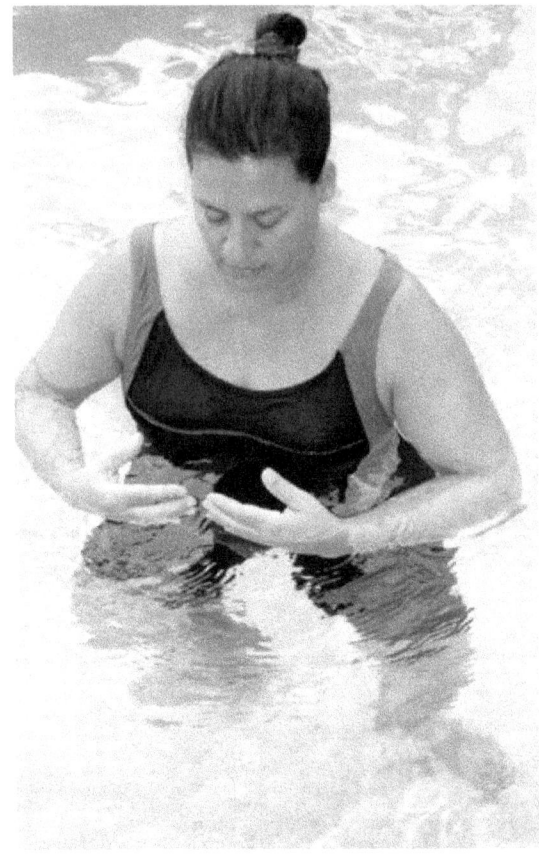 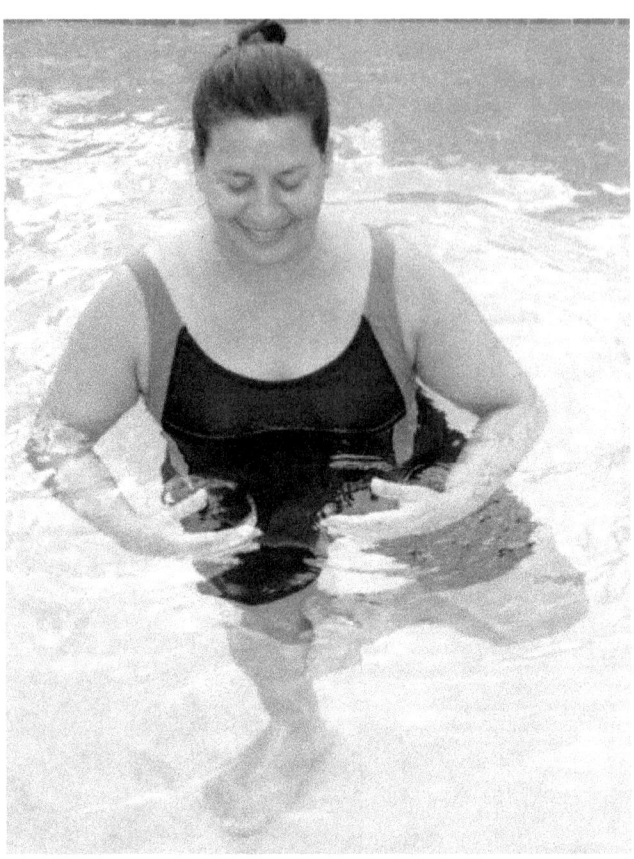

1   **2**

Begin this exercise in the starting position as listed in the previous exercise and shown again in Diagram 1.

Inhale and bend your left knee out to the side of your body and place the bottom of your left foot on the inside of your right leg just above the knee. Hold it there and breathe in and out slowly and without effort.

You may find that it is very difficult to keep your balance against the natural current of the water. Do your best.

When finished, release the foot to the starting position and repeat this exercise on the other side of your body by bending your right knee and placing the bottom of your right foot on the inside of your left leg.

NOTE: The higher up the leg you place your foot, the harder the exercise will become.

Balance Continued

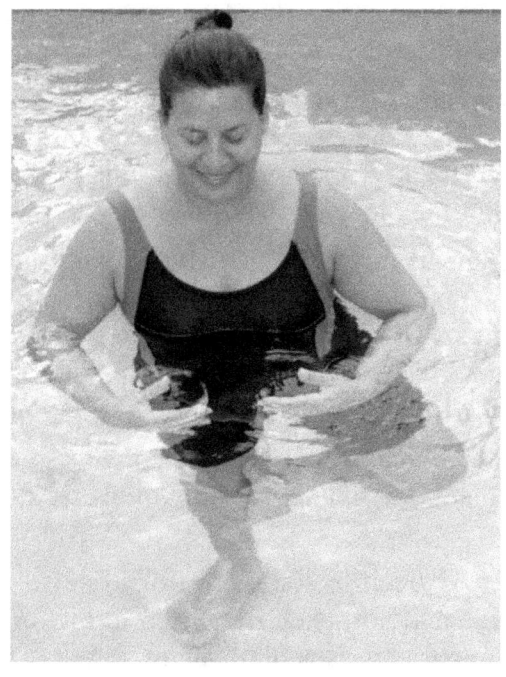 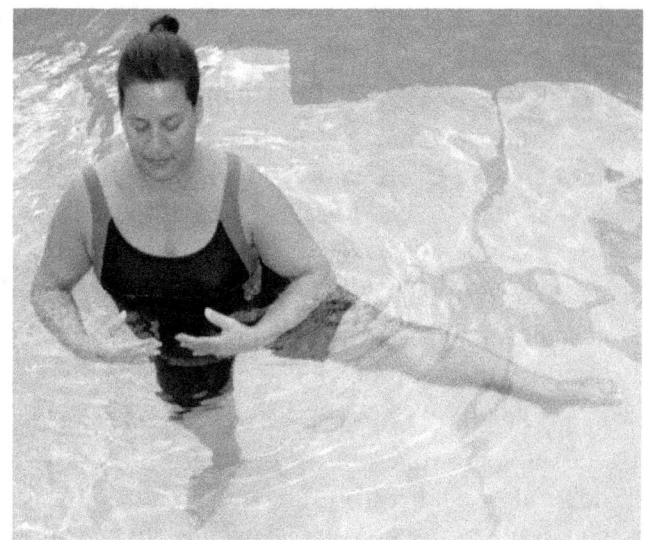

1   2

If you found the previous balance exercise too easy for you, then you might want to try this on instead.

Begin this exercise in the starting position as listed previously. Bend your left knee out to the side of your body and place the bottom of your right foot on the inside of your right leg.

Inhale and find your balance and as you exhale extend your left leg straight out to the side of your body with your toes pointed.

Breathe in and out naturally as you hold this pose (shown in Diagram #2) and find your balance within the water. Bend your left knee and return the foot to the right leg as shown in Diagram #1. Return to starting position and repeat this exercise on the other side of your body by bending your right knee and placing the bottom of your right foot on the inside of your left leg and while exhaling, extend your right leg straight out from the side of your body keeping your toes pointed. Hold the position breathing naturally in and out. Find the balance within the currents of the water and then release.

Cool Down

Cool Downs are a series of movements that are used after an exercise class as a means to return the heart rate back to its normal pre-exercise rate. The more you exercise, the stronger your heart will become and the shorter the period of time it will take for the heart rate to return to normal.

Many first time exercisers will experience a prolong lapse of time where their heart rate may remain in an elevated state. This is why it is suggested for first time exercisers not to over due their first exercise class. If you are a first time exerciser, then you should work at your own fitness level and not 'push' through exercises after you have become winded or fatigued.

When just beginning your first month of workouts, maybe just try each exercise once and then finish for the day. Chart your body's progress as to how sore your muscles feel the next day. If completing all the exercises in this book at one time is too much for you, then pick one exercise for the ankles, one exercise for the legs, etc. and then just do those exercises for a week, or month, as the case may be. You could then add, or trade out, the exercises for the following workout period.

It makes no sense to tax your body's energy system by doing exercises to the point of soreness, exhaustion, or injury. For us, maintaining a healthy and strong body should be a top priority. After all, this is the only body we have; we should be kind to it.

So set some time out of your very busy day to treat yourself to some form of exercise. Even sitting down in a chair or on the couch, and doing the ankle and arm exercises listed in this book is better than doing nothing. You can even perform some of these exercises while lying in bed.

If you need help in adapting any of these exercises to your own specific limitations, just drop me an email at FrancineMilford@verizon.net and we can discuss options.

Cool Down

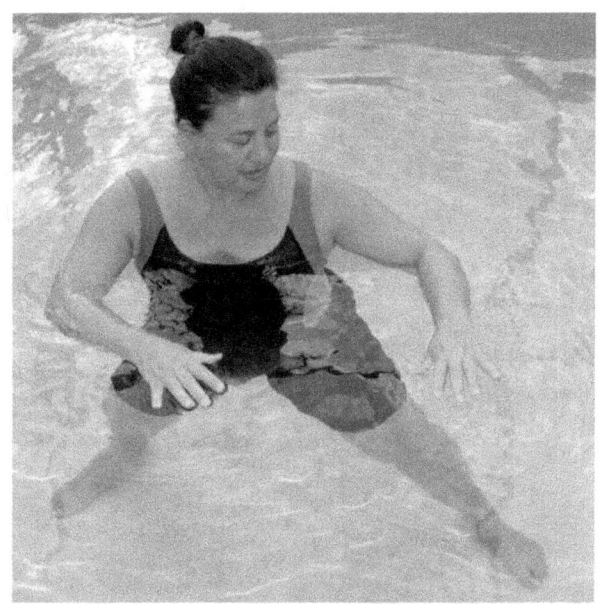

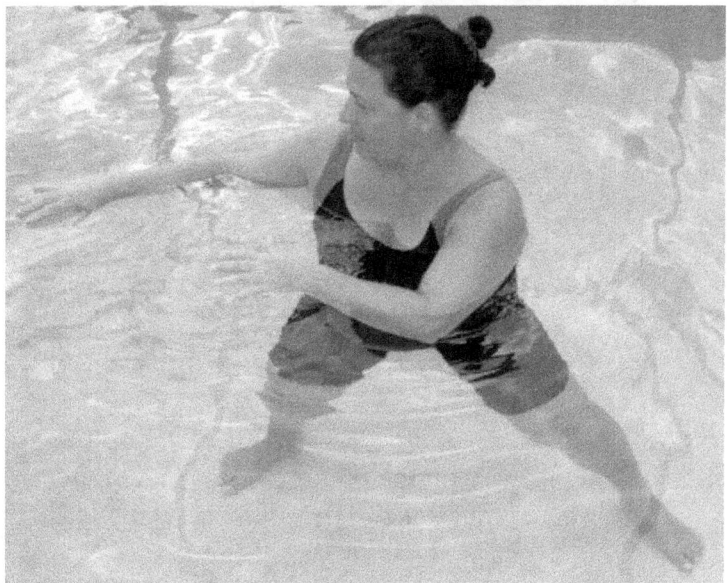

You can add mindfulness and Breathwork to this cool down exercise. To do this exercise, spread your legs apart as far as you comfortably can to maintain your body's balance in the water.

Place your hands, palm down, at the very top of the water and pretend that there are flower petals floating on the top of the water. Gently push the flower petals to the left and then to right trying not to disturb the petals, or the water.

As you perform this exercise, breathe in as slowly and deeply as you can. Make your movements as slow and deliberate as you can. Do this exercise for as long as you like, and enjoy.

The Qi Ball

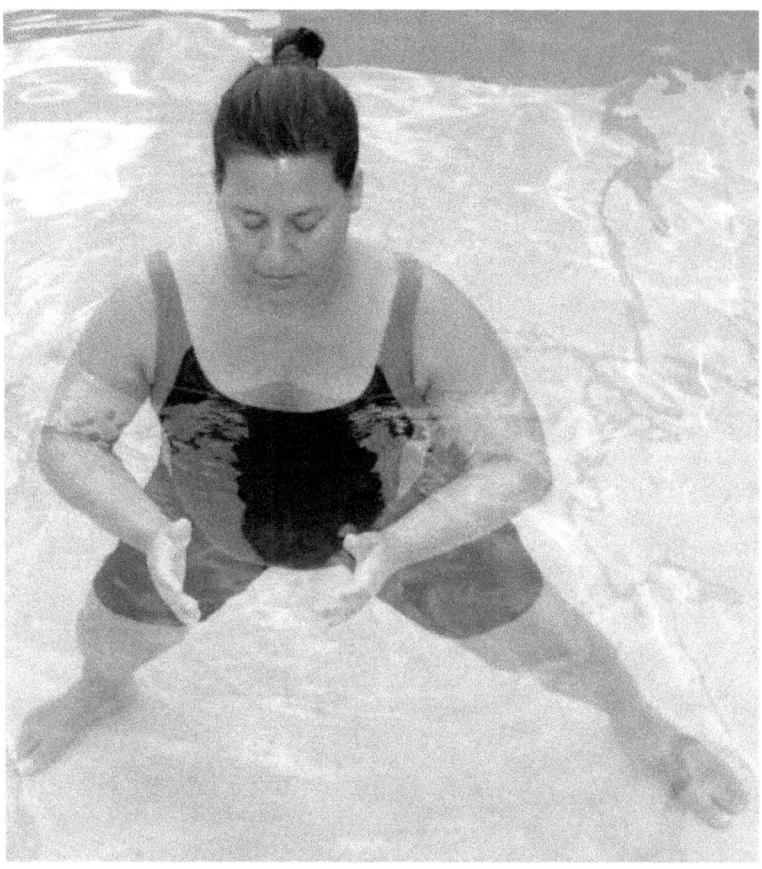

Now that you have allowed your body to cool down after your exercise session, you should be feeling very good at this point.

Stand with your feet firmly planted on the bottom of the pool. You can keep your feet together or apart at any width you desire where you can keep your balance easily in the water.

Bring both of your hands up in front of your body at heart level (should be just under the water line) with palms facing each other. Inhale and pull the hands away from each other to about 1-2' apart. When you exhale, bring the hands towards each other to about 6-12" apart. Continue inhaling and exhaling in the way for as long as you enjoy this exercise.

Chapter Six

The Old Food Guide Pyramid 2005

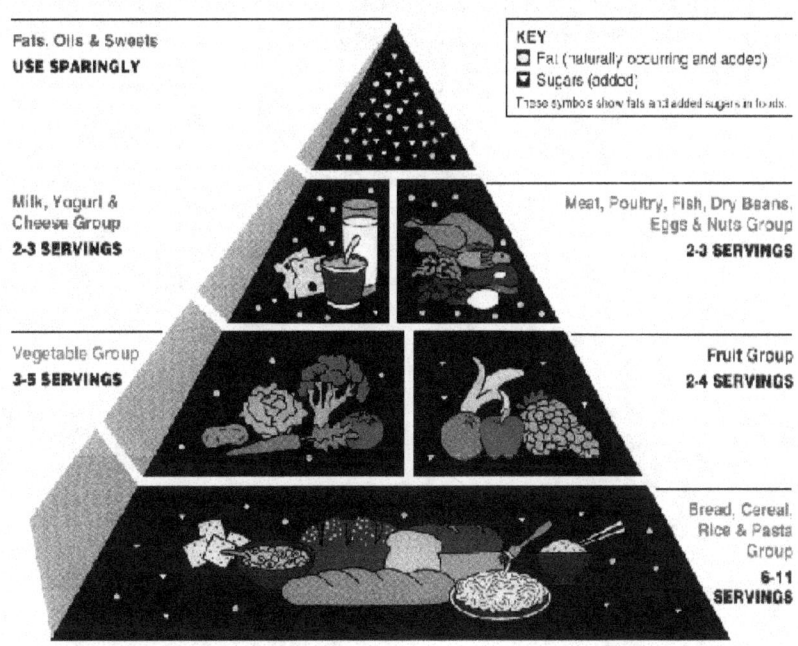

The above Food Guide Pyramid was developed by the U. S. Department of Agriculture. It is a guide to food choices that we should be making every day in order to maintain a healthy diet. It is a guideline as to what daily choices we should be making for ourselves to ensure that we receiving the nutrients and calories that we need to maintain a healthy weight.

A typical day would include 6-11 servings of bread, cereal, rice, and pasta. Add to that 3-5 servings of Vegetables, 2-4 servings of fruit, 2-3 servings of meat, poultry, dry beans, eggs, or nuts and 2 to 3 servings of milk, yogurt or cheese. The only restrictions on this pyramid are to use fats, oils and sweet sparingly.

To see how well you are faring in feeding your body, write down everything you ate in one day, from waking up in the morning to going to bed at night. Yes, that includes how many teaspoons of sugar you put in your coffee and how many pads of butter you put on your biscuits.

Don't make any judgments (yet) on what you are writing down. Just jot down every morsel for one day. What you see staring back at you is a true mirror of what is going on in your body. Your daily diet will give you many clues as to your moods and experiences through the day.

Be sure to add the time you are eating every delectable morsel. You will soon learn a lot about yourself and may answer many of the questions you have as to why you are always tired.

If are not sure what constitutes a serving, then check the writing on the box, bag, or can. This information is always listed on the label on the product.

If you find yourself eating more than 1 serving, then be sure to count that as 2, or 3, servings. Actual serving sizes may surprise you as to how small they really are. When you start measuring out what constituents a serving size and see how many calories go with every serving size, you are on your way to making intelligent choices for your health.

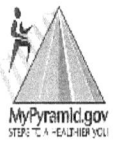

Sample Menus for a 2000 Calorie Food Pattern

Averaged over a week, this seven day menu provides all of the recommended amounts of nutrients and food from each food group. (Italicized foods are part of the dish or food that preceeds it.)

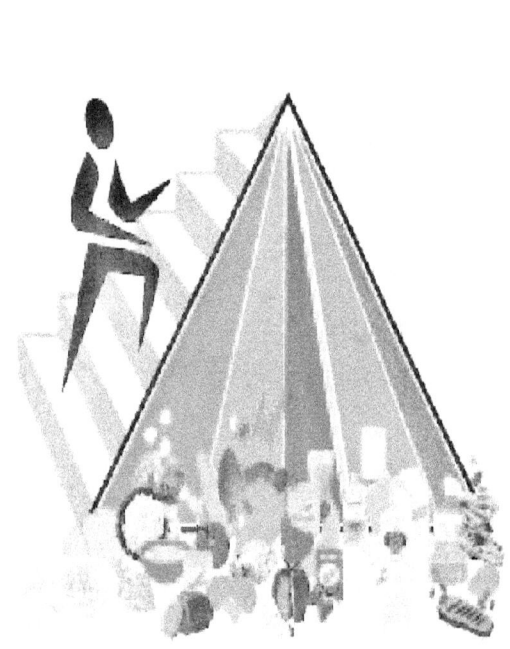

Food Group	Daily Average
GRAINS	Total Grains (oz eq) 6.0
	Whole Grains 3.4
	Refined Grains 2.6
VEGETABLES*	Total Veg* (cups) 2.6
FRUITS	Fruits (cups) 2.1
MILK	Milk (cups) 3.1
MEAT & BEANS	Meat/Beans (oz eq) 5.6
OILS	Oils (tsp/grams) 7.2 tsp/32.4 g

Nutrient	Daily Average
Calories	1994
Protein, g	98
Protein, % kcal	20
Carbohydrate, g	264
Carbohydrate, % kcal	53
Total fat, g	67
Total fat, % kcal	30
Saturated fat, g	16
Saturated fat, % kcal	7.0
Monounsaturated fat, g	23
Polyunsaturated fat, g	23
Linoleic Acid, g	21
Alpha-linolenic Acid, g	1.1
Cholesterol, mg	207
Total dietary fiber, g	31
Potassium, mg	4715
Sodium, mg*	1948
Calcium, mg	1389
Magnesium, mg	432
Copper, mg	1.9
Iron, mg	21
Phosphorus, mg	1830
Zinc, mg	14
Thiamin, mg	1.9
Riboflavin, mg	2.5
Niacin Equivalents, mg	24
Vitamin B6, mg	2.9
Vitamin B12, mcg	18.4
Vitamin C, mg	190
Vitamin E, mg (AT)	18.9
Vitamin A, mcg (RAE)	1430
Dietary Folate Equivalents, mcg	558

*Vegetable subgroups	(weekly totals)
Dk-Green Veg (cups)	3.3
Orange Veg (cups)	2.3
Beans/ Peas (cups)	3.0
Starchy Veg (cups)	3.4
Other Veg (cups)	6.6

* Starred items are foods that are labelled as no-salt-added, low-sodium, or low-salt versions of the foods. They can also be prepared from scratch with little or no added salt. All other foods are regular commercial products which contain variable levels of sodium. Average sodium level of the 7 day menu assumes no-salt-added in cooking or at the table.

For a free color, downloadable chart of your own, as shown above, please go to: www.MyPyramid.gov . The site also contains free downloadable information on starting a healthy diet, what constitutes a serving, and sample menu charts. The site also contains resource material for those in the health care industry for to share with your clients. The recommendations listed are based on the Dietary Guidelines for Americans in 2005. The guidelines are recommended for the general public over the age of 2.

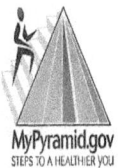

MyPyramid Worksheet

Check how you did today and set a goal to aim for tomorrow

MyPyramid.gov
STEPS TO A HEALTHIER YOU

Write in Your Choices for Today	Food Group	Tip	Goal	List each food choice in its food group*	Estimate Your Total
_____ _____ _____ _____	GRAINS	Make at least half your grains whole grains	**6 ounce equivalents** (1 ounce equivalent is about 1 slice bread, 1 cup dry cereal, or ½ cup rice or pasta)	_____ _____ _____	_____ ounce equivalents
_____ _____ _____ _____	VEGETABLES	Try to have vegetables from several subgroups each day	**2 ½ cups** Subgroups: Dark Green, Orange, Starchy, Dry Beans and Peas, Other Veggies	_____ _____ _____	_____ cups
_____ _____ _____	FRUITS	Make most choices fruit, not juice	**2 cups**	_____ _____	_____ cups
_____ _____ _____	MILK	Choose fat-free or low fat most often	**3 cups** (1 ½ ounces cheese = 1 cup milk)	_____ _____	_____ cups
_____ _____ _____	MEAT & BEANS	Choose lean meat and poultry. Vary your choices—more fish, beans, peas, nuts, and seeds	**5 ½ ounce equivalents** (1 ounce equivalent is 1 ounce meat, poultry or fish, 1 T. peanut butter, ½ ounce nuts, ¼ cup dry beans or peas)	_____ _____	_____ ounce equivalents
_____ _____ _____	PHYSICAL ACTIVITY	Build more physical activity into your daily routine at home and work.	At least **30 minutes** of moderate to vigorous activity a day, 10 minutes or more at a time.	*Some foods don't fit into any group. These "extras" may be mainly fat or sugar—limit your intake of these.	_____ minutes

How did you do today? ☐ Great   ☐ So-So   ☐ Not so Great

My food goal for tomorrow is: _____

My activity goal for tomorrow is: _____

79

MyPyramid Food Intake Pattern Calorie Levels

MyPyramid assigns Individuals to a calorie level based on their sex, age, and activity level.

The chart below identifies the calorie levels for males and females by age and activity level. Calorie levels are provided for each year of childhood, from 2-18 years, and for adults in 5-year increments.

	MALES				FEMALES		
Activity level	Sedentary*	Mod. active*	Active*	**Activity level**	Sedentary*	Mod. active*	Active*
AGE				**AGE**			
2	1000	1000	1000	2	1000	1000	1000
3	1000	1400	1400	3	1000	1200	1400
4	1200	1400	1600	4	1200	1400	1400
5	1200	1400	1600	5	1200	1400	1600
6	1400	1600	1800	6	1200	1400	1600
7	1400	1600	1800	7	1200	1600	1800
8	1400	1600	2000	8	1400	1600	1800
9	1600	1800	2000	9	1400	1600	1800
10	1600	1800	2200	10	1400	1800	2000
11	1800	2000	2200	11	1600	1800	2000
12	1800	2200	2400	12	1600	2000	2200
13	2000	2200	2600	13	1600	2000	2200
14	2000	2400	2800	14	1800	2000	2400
15	2200	2600	3000	15	1800	2000	2400
16	2400	2800	3200	16	1800	2000	2400
17	2400	2800	3200	17	1800	2000	2400
18	2400	2800	3200	18	1800	2000	2400
19-20	2600	2800	3000	19-20	2000	2200	2400
21-25	2400	2800	3000	21-25	2000	2200	2400
26-30	2400	2600	3000	26-30	1800	2000	2400
31-35	2400	2600	3000	31-35	1800	2000	2200
36-40	2400	2600	2800	36-40	1800	2000	2200
41-45	2200	2600	2800	41-45	1800	2000	2200
46-50	2200	2400	2800	46-50	1800	2000	2200
51-55	2200	2400	2800	51-55	1600	1800	2200
56-60	2200	2400	2600	56-60	1600	1800	2200
61-65	2000	2400	2600	61-65	1600	1800	2000
66-70	2000	2200	2600	66-70	1600	1800	2000
71-75	2000	2200	2600	71-75	1600	1800	2000
76 and up	2000	2200	2400	76 and up	1600	1800	2000

*Calorie levels are based on the Estimated Energy Requirements (EER) and activity levels from the Institute of Medicine Dietary Reference Intakes Macronutrients Report, 2002.
SEDENTARY = less than 30 minutes a day of moderate physical activity in addition to daily activities.
MOD. ACTIVE = at least 30 minutes up to 60 minutes a day of moderate physical activity in addition to daily activities.
ACTIVE = 60 or more minutes a day of moderate physical activity in addition to daily activities.

United StatesDepartment of Agriculture
Center for Nutrition Policy and Promotion
April 2005
CNPP-XX

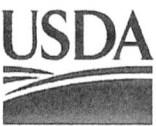

About the Author

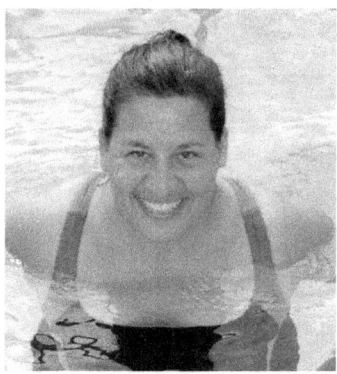

Francine Milford is a licensed massage therapist, personal trainer and owner of the Reiki Center of Venice. She has had a very long career in the Fitness Industry. Working for more than twenty years in a variety of sports and exercise related classes, Francine is also an avid walker and enjoys reading a book audio tape while bicycling around the neighborhood.

She has achieved certifications through the YMCA S.A.F.E. Aerobic Program, AEA Aquatics Exercise Association, ESA Exercise Safety Association, and AFAA Aerobics Fitness Association.

Francine has also received the Tai Chi for Arthritis Certification having studied under Dr. Paul Lam, as well as, 180 hours of professional training in Tai Kwan Do.

She has taught such classes as Kick Boxing, Bench Stepping, Low Impact Aerobics, High Impact Aerobics, Basic Floor and Senior Aerobics and all types of Water Aerobic classes.

As a personal trainer and fitness specialist, Francine has been hired to lead classes and workshops at offices, condo organizations, clubs and private groups.

Having spent the last ten years working with the senior population, Francine has developed exercises that are both safe and effective for those with physical limitations.

Francine has authored more than 35 books that are available at www.lulu.com/Francine, www.amazon.com, and at the www.ReikiCenterofVenice.com, and www.FrancineMilford.com

You can write to Francine at her office at the Reiki Center of Venice, 101 W. Venice Ave., Suite 31-7, Venice, Fl. 34285 or by email at FrancineMilford@verizon.net

If you enjoyed this book than you may also enjoy the second in the H2O Workout series titled, H2O Workouts: Using your Poodle Noodle.

Book Titles by Francine Milford

Tuning Fork Therapy® Levels One-Seven Manual

Tuning Fork Therapy® Planetary Forks

Tuning Fork Therapy® Accessing your Energy Body

Tuning Fork Therapy®: How to Make a Gem Elixir

Tuning Fork Therapy®: Blood Pressure

Tuning Fork Therapy®: Using Tuning Forks in Water

Tuning Fork Therapy® Dog's Chakras

Tuning Fork Therapy® Cat's Chakras

Tuning Fork Therapy® Dog's Acupoints

Hand Therapy for Computer Users

Makko Ho: Six Exercises for Health and Well Being

DoIn: A form of self massage

Usui Reiki, Levels One Manual

Usui Reiki, Level Two Manual

Usui Reiki, Master Level

Usui Reiki: A Mother's Journey to Health and Healing

Aroma~Care: How to make your own Perfume

Aroma~Care: Make your own Magical Blends

Aroma~Care: Pet Aromatherapy

H2OWorkouts: Basic Moves and Using your Pool Noodle

Copper Wands: Levels One-Seven Manual

For a complete and up-to-date list of other book titles, please visit publisher at www.lulu.com/Francine.

References

American College of Sport Medicine, Guidelines for Graded Exercise Testing and Exercise Prescription. Philadelphia: Lea and Febiger, 1995.

American Red Cross, Swimming and Diving, 1992.

Aqua Fitness, The low-impact total body workout, Mimi Rodriguwq Adamia, DK Publishing, Inc., 2002.

Aquatic Exercise Association, ESA, Aquatic Concepts, a Resource Manual for Aquatic Fitness Instructors, 1990.

Beasley, Bob L., et al. "Metabolic and Heart Rate Responses to Aquatic Exercise," Research Council Proceedings-Southern District, American Alliance of Health, Physical Education, Recreation and Dance, 1987.

Conrad, Casey C. "The New Aqua Dynamics: Water Exercise to Fit Any Body. Alexandria, Va., National Spa and Pool Institute, 1985.

Fitness Aquatics, LeAnne Case, 1997.

Frangolias, D.D., and Rhodes, E.C. "Metabolic Responses and Mechanisms during Water Immersion Running and Exercise." Sports Medicine, 22 (1) (1996).

Hoeger, W.W.K. Principles and Labs for Physical Fitness and Wellness. Englewood, CO: Morton Publishing, 1999.

Water Aerobics for Fitness & Wellnes, Second Edition, Terry-Ann Spitzer Gibson and Werner W. K. Hoeger.

NOTES:

www.ingramcontent.com/pod-product-compliance
Lightning Source LLC
Chambersburg PA
CBHW052007280526
45793CB00005B/881